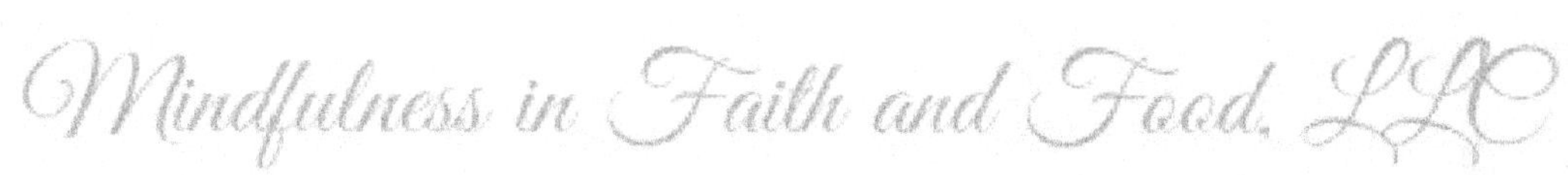

Thank you for purchasing The Nourishing Meal Builder!

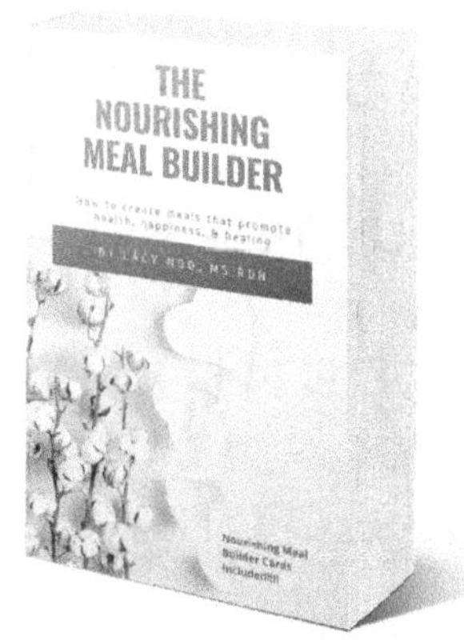

As a gift to you, here is a 25% off coupon code for any other Mindfulness in Faith and Food, LLC eboooks: THANKYOU25

You are also invited to become a member of the Mindful Family for FREE! You can join here!

As memebers, you will receive:

- The FREE 7-day Mindful Planner
- The FREE Random Acts of KIndness Planner
- The FREE Mindful Lunchbox Notes
- The FREE Healthy Lunchbox Checklist and More!

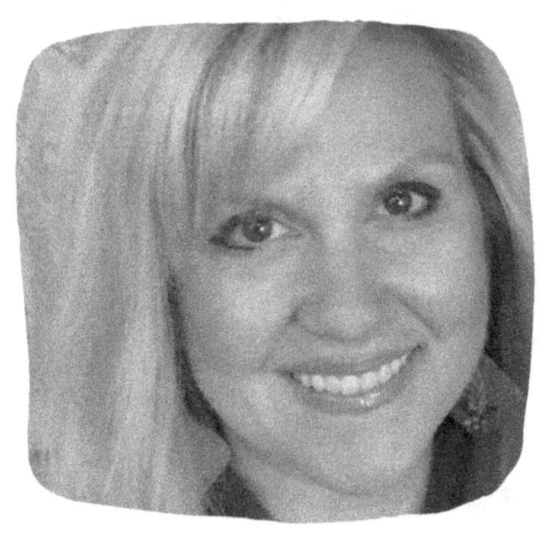

Lacy Ngo is a registered dietitian with a Masters in Human Nutrition. Lacy is the owner of Mindfulness in Faith and Food, LLC and Mindful Vending. Mindfulness in Faith and Food is a faith-based nutrition website that focuses on mindful eating AND mindful living. Mindful Vending is a dietitian owned and operated healthy vending company. Whether it's through her blog or through her healthy vending machine snacks, Lacy's goal is to provide tips and snacks that will make healthy eating easier and more convenient for busy families living in a choatic world.

www.mindfulnessinfaithandfood.com

Affiliate Disclosure

This book may contain affiliate links. If you click on one of my affiliate links and make a purchase, I may receive a small commission. This comes at no additional cost to you. I only recommend products that I use and love!

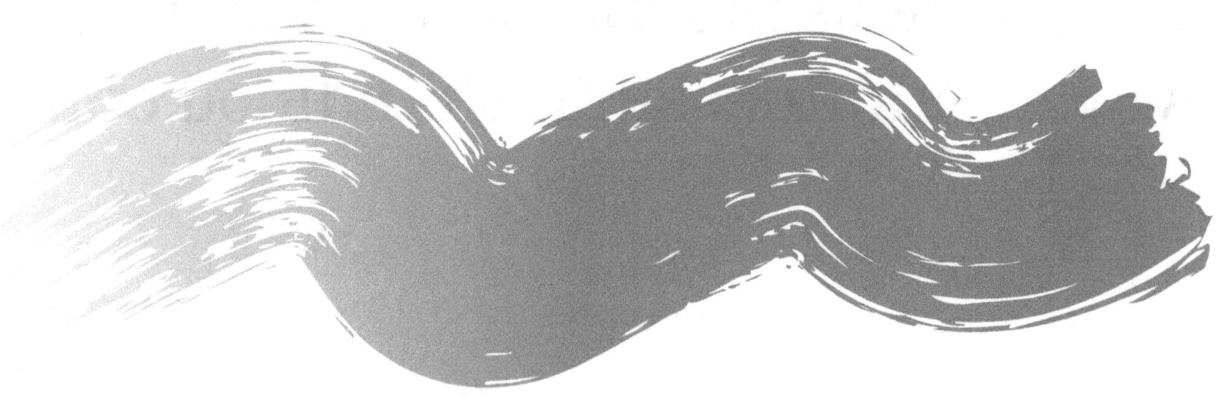

www.mindfulnessinfaithandfood.com

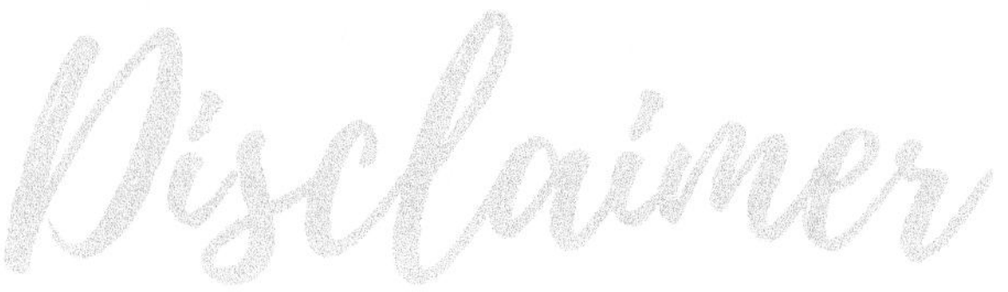

Disclaimer

This book does not replace medical advice. This book contains general nutrition information from a registered dietitian; however, nutritional needs vary among individuals based on labs, medical conditions, genetics, etc. Please discuss any medical conditions one-on-one with a doctor and/or dietitian. A dietitian can help you personalize a diet for any specific conditions. For example, if you have diabetes, a dietitian can tailor diet recommendations specifically to your condition. This site is not liable or responsible if someone takes advice from this book and has any problems.

ACKNOWLEDEMENTS

To my Family; Chad, Hilt, & Neeshie,

You give me my inspiration and my drive. My desire to write this book came from my desire to have the energy and time to be a good mom and wife to you.

 I thank God for you. Being your mom and wife has taught me about how to live a happier, healthier, and more purposeful life.

Love,

Lacy

Table of Contents

Chapter 1
Why This Book & Why These Foods

If you have read any of my blog posts or my last book, you know I am all about easy, convenient, NOURISHING meals that help me (and you) live a healthy, happy, and meaningful life. I don't want to just live though, I want to thrive AND have the energy to love and help others to the best of my ability. And I wish the same for you.

So how does the strategy in this book help me and you live your healthiest, happiest, most meaningful life?

This book can help in two big ways:

1. Provide **Nutrients** that help you feel your best, have energy, and thrive. (i.e. Provide nutrients to help you live your healthiest, happiest, most meaningful life.)
2. Provide a quick and easy way to get these nourishing foods on the table everyday.

Let's really dive into reason number 1:

Provide Nutrients that help you live your healthiest, happiest, most meaningful life

God gave us the gift of food. Food brings us joy and has life-sustaining powers, and yet nutrition can be so confusing…

Sometimes we may want to eat these nourishing foods, but we have so many questions:

- Which foods do what?
- What foods are anti-inflammatory?
- Are there foods that boost the immune system?
- What foods help with mood, depression, anxiety, and brain function?
- Can certain foods boost memory and reduce the risk of Alzheimer's and dementia?
- What foods reduce the risk of heart disease, cancer, stroke and diabetes?
- What foods help with bloating, stomach distention, constipation, GERD, cramps, diarrhea, or other stomach problems?
- Can certain foods reduce joint pain, arthritis pain, headaches, and migraines?
- Are there foods that can help with autoimmune or neurodegenerative diseases?

- And can I find a list of all of these foods that can do all of these things in one spot?...
- And is there a stress-free easy way to make sure I am getting all of these foods in my daily diet?

· ·

About a year ago, I got into a funk about my kids getting older. For about two weeks, I cried every night. A few weeks later, I developed a bad cough and had so much mucus in my stomach that I kept throwing up mucus and food. It was so severe that I couldn't do much of anything except lie in the bed and throw up. This lasted for about two weeks!!!!

I finally felt better after my doctor started me on a steroid, but two weeks later I came down with the same symptoms again!

Being a dietitian, I began thinking, "maybe it's something I'm eating? Maybe I'm sensitive to a certain food or maybe my gut bacteria are out of balance?" I knew certain foods could affect mood, inflammation, and immunity; so I decided to be intentional about what foods I was eating....

I wanted to make sure I was eating food EVERY week that promoted a healthy mood, gut, and immune system. But… why stop there?

Yes, I wanted to make a list of foods that could help improve MY specific symptoms, but I thought, 'I want more. I want to make a list of nutrients and foods that can reduce the risk or Dementia, Alzheimer's, Cancer, and stomach problems like cramps, stomach distention, and diarrhea. I want to include nutrients and foods in this list that can help reduce the risk of strokes, heart disease, and even autoimmune diseases.

I wanted a COMPLETE list all in one place.

So I decided to make one. For the past year, I have been developing a database of nutrients that are astoundingly beneficial to our bodies in a multitude of ways…

What if I told you that there are foods you can eat that can help alleviate symptoms and/or GREATLY reduce your risk of developing MANY conditions like:

- Heat Disease, Stroke
- Diabetes
- Inflammation
- Cancer
- Rheumatoid Arthritis & Joint Pain
- Fibromyalgia
- Distention
- Bloating
- IBS & IBD
- Leaky Gut
- Heartburn & GERD
- Migraines & Headaches
- Diarrhea, Constipation, Stomach Pain, Gas, and Cramps
- Fatigue/Decrease Energy Levels
- Frequent Colds and Illnesses, Mucus Drainage and Phlegm
- Autoimmune diseases
- Allergies
- Memory problems, Cognitive Decline, Poor Cognitive focus, Alzheimer's, & Dementia
- Hormone imbalance
- Mood disorders like depression, anxiety, and stress
- Acne
- Insomnia
- Inability to lose weight
- ADHD (Symptoms)
- Autism (Symptoms)
- Small Intestine Bacteria Overgrowth
- Crohn's Disease
- Lupus
- Ulcerative Colitis

Many foods can alleviate disease symptoms or are linked to reducing the risk of developing these diseases and conditions. Many of these links are backed by extensive studies while some are in the first stages of research. Either way, these foods are healthy for your body.

You are probably not surprised to know that often the same foods that improve mood and support immunity are the same foods that help reduce the risk of all those diseases like Alzheimer's, cancer, and heart disease. Moreover, the foods found to increase the risk of one of those diseases increases the risk of almost all the other conditions on the list as well.

In fact, I was able to come up with a list of nutrients I wanted to make sure my family was eating every week based on research.

So How does all of this relate back to purpose number 1, which is to provide nourishing goods so that we can live our healthiest, happiest, most meaningful life?

You see, my goals in life are to serve God and others and love the people around me the best I can. (When you really think about it, these are probably the goals for many of us.**)**

Eating foods from God's earth that nourish my mind, body, and soul can help me get closer to these goals.

So my hope for this books is to provide a list of foods that:

- Promote health and provide energy to serve God and others;

-Fuel our minds to learn,

-Promote a positive mood. (Although we should strive to show kindness no matter what, showing kindness is a much harder when we are hurting ourselves. This is 100% true for me.)

Does Nutrition *REALLY* have that Big of an Impact?

I selected these particular nutrients because the research backs them up. The MIND, Mediterranean, and Blue Zone diets as well as Gut healthy foods, ALL contain these nutrients. All these diets have been shown to reduce the risk of a multitude of diseases and conditions. Moreover, the studies that were done on each individual nutrient on the list show the same benefits.

So below are just a few small samples of what others are saying about the overwhelming amount of research (Find a large list of references at the end of this book):

According to Marilyn Haugen and Doug Cook, RD in 175 *Best Superfood Blender Recipes*, "A diet rich in fruits, vegetables, nuts, seeds, legumes, whole grains, fish, antioxidants, and healthy herbs and spices can reduce the risk of Type 2 diabetes by 90% and Alzheimer's by 40%!!!!" These foods are the cornerstones of the Mediterranean, MIND, Blue Zone, and gut healthy diets, and these foods mentioned by Haugen and Cook are, of course, the main foods featured in this book.

According to the Pharmaceutical Research Journal, 90-95% of cancer has a root cause in environmental and lifestyle factors, with 25-30% due to tobacco and 30-35% linked to diet.

The Mediterranean Diet

Maggie Moon talks about both the Mediterranean and MIND diet in her book, The MIND Diet. In her book, Moon states, "…studies have shown that Mediterranean-style eating patterns are linked with lower risk of neurodegenerative diseases like Parkinson's and now the MIND diet has been shown to protect against cognitive decline in aging." Evidence also suggests that the Mediterranean diet may be beneficial for many, many other conditions like mood disorders, ADHD, cancer, asthma, and even seasonal allergies.

MIND Diet

Based on the research, I can concur with Maggie Moon when she writes, "The two key MIND diet studies show how the diet keeps the aging brain seven and a half years younger and reduces the risk of developing Alzheimer's disease by 53%."

Blue Zone Foods

In business, we look to the businesses who are getting it right and try to follow their lead. We use the term benchmark to refer to something that serves as a standard best practice. Perhaps we should do this with nutrition as well. Are there areas where people seem to be getting this "living a healthy life" thing right? Maybe we should see what they are doing and try to incorporate some of their practices into our lives. Turns out we already have our "healthy living" benchmark. We call these areas the Blue Zones.

The Blue Zone research is a bit different. The Blue Zone refers to areas in the world where people are living long, high-quality lives. The people living in these 5 Blue Zones have lower rates of chronic disease and have reported a higher satisfaction with their quality of life and well-being. The 5 regions where you can find the world's longest living people who are living without significant memory or physical problems are:

- Loma Linda, California
- Ikaria, Greece
- Okinawa, Japan
- Nicoya, Costa Rica
- Sardina, Italy

So, what are these Blue Zone guys and gals doing that the rest of us aren't?

These Blue Zone inhabitants share several common characteristics.

First, their diets are 90-100% plant based. There diets are mostly beans, legumes, fruits, vegetables, whole grains, and nuts. They also eat small amounts or fish, lean meats, and eggs; and the most common oil used in the Blue Zones is olive oil. They eat foods that contain natural sugar, but rarely eat foods that contain added sugar or are heavily processed. Fermented vegetables are common in the Blue Zone areas. They mainly drink water, but also drink coffee, tea, and small amounts of red wine.

And yep, you guessed it. These foods are prominent in *The Nourishing Meal Builder.*

Gut Health

Take that list of medical conditions from earlier and duplicate it here. Although some of the research is preliminary, gut health, alone, has been linked to almost all of the previously listed conditions.

But what is a healthy gut? A healthy gut has more good bacteria than bad bacteria and is also digesting and absorbing properly. Inversely, a leaky gut is not absorbing properly. With a leaky gut, the wrong things, like undigested foods and bacteria are leaking from the gut into your blood stream.

Dietitian, Dianne Rishikof writes in her ebook, *Health Takes Guts*, "The influence that gut microbes have cannot be overstated. They are the root cause and solutions to most health troubles."

Kara Lydon, RDN writes in *Nourish your Namaste*, "We are learning more and more about the importance of gut health. Gut health not only affects digestion, but also the immune system, weight, mood, allergies, food sensitivities, and autoimmune disease."

Lydon also writes, "Solid research shows that higher intakes of heavily processed foods, refined sugars, sodium, and saturated fat can negatively impact the immune system."

According to dietitian, Ali Miller, in her book *The Anti-Anxiety Diet,* "Learning about leaky gut and its role in driving inflammation throughout the body as well as driving autism, ADHD, anxiety, bipolar disorder, dyslexia, and depression, was mind-blowing!"

Also in *The Anti-Anxiety Diet*, Miller states, "…addressing anxiety and improving the status of your gut can greatly enhance the function of your brain, and ultimately, your entire body."

Inflammation

Based on a study published in the Journal of the American College of Cardiology, diets high in refined starches, sugar, and trans fats and low in fruits, vegetables, whole grains, and omega-3 fatty acids appear to be pro-inflammatory, and diets rich in whole foods; including healthful carbohydrates, fats, and protein sources; are anti-inflammatory in nature.

There is a large amount of substantial research on the foods and nutrients listed in this book. In the reference section, you will find a huge list of research articles that discuss the Mediterranean diet, MIND diet, gut health, individual nutrients as well as how specific food, nutrients and diets relate to specific medical conditions. Please feel free to look up these studies on your own. They are absolutely fascinating and exciting.

Real Stories

As dietitian's we know it's important to focus on the research and not the anecdotal evidence (i.e. testimonies). I agree with this and yet many of us are not convinced to alter our habits until we hear someone else's story. I totally get it. When we hear someone's story, it becomes more real, doesn't it? When we see someone's life improved dramatically, the impact is seen firsthand. Stories are so much more relatable than all those numbers and percentages from research. So now that we have established the research is there, let's talk about a couple of real people and case studies.

First, let's go back to my story. I was truly sad about my kids getting older. Food didn't change that. My youngest had started kindergarten so those painful feelings were real, but how quickly they came and the fact that they were not going away, made me feel like something else was going on in my body that exasperated those feelings.

Then, when around the same time the excessive mucus just wouldn't go away either, I decided to add some gut healing, mood enhancing foods to my diet. I started intentionally eating more mood enhancing foods and probiotics every day and my sadness and mucus WENT away! Plus, I have always had severe stop-you-in-your-tracks seasonal allergies. They would hit like clockwork every fall and spring. Then I made these dietary changes, and for the first time...ever, spring came, and the allergies, didn't.

This was unprecedented, but would it happen again? Yep, in the fall following these diet changes, my allergies were minimal and short-lived. Even my husband commented. He had gotten use to me being sick for two weeks every spring and fall. When it didn't happen, he was shocked and relieved for me. We have been married 15 years, and this was the first time my allergies didn't do me in for weeks!

 Moreover, I have always (since middle school) had to go to a dermatologist for acne. I was 37 with acne problems.

Once I was more intentional about the foods I put into my body, the acne almost completely went away!!! Was it a coincidence? I truly don't know, that is why looking at the research is so important too!

I want to take my story back a little further to when my son had something called Bronchiectasis. Bronchiectasis is basically damaged lungs. His became damaged due to a case of pneumonia (brought on by the common cold). Because of his condition, he had to continuously be on antibiotics 3 days a week. This was ongoing, meaning he was not supposed to stop taking antibiotics ever. Even on antibiotics, his lungs kept having problems. The doctors finally decided it was time to remove one of my son's lobes.

Removing the lobe was a success, and he no longer has bronchiectasis. But about two months after his surgery, he was diagnosed with a seemingly unrelated autoimmune disease called HSP. When you have HSP your blood vessels leak, which can cause all kinds of scary problems. He is now in remission, and for many, HSP never comes back.

So what does this all have to do with nutrition? Maybe nothing. Maybe there is no explanation, but I do know that poor gut health is linked to autoimmune diseases. And although the relationship of HSP and gut health has not been studied, HSP is an autoimmune disease. Although antibiotics kill the bad bacteria, antibiotics can also kill the good bacteria too. So perhaps my son began to have a gut imbalance due to being on antibiotics. Per my own knowledge and doctors advice, I made sure my son was eating a probiotic everyday while he was on an antibiotic. Still, it may not have been enough to stop the gut imbalance.

I am not sure if this was a contributor to my son's HSP, but I do know that I am much more conscious about what my son eats now. I encourage him and my daughter to eat foods that support the immune system and promote a healthy gut. After all, his pneumonia developed from a common cold virus so strengthening the immune system is now a priority!

Finally, my son has always had issues with anxiety as well. (I'm sure his medical issues have contributed to his anxious personality). So I also began encouraging him to eat foods that may help with mood and anxiety, and guess what?!? I have seen a big difference in his mood and behavior!

If you want to read some really cool, like-give-you-chills God Moment stories related to my son's illnesses, you can find them on my blog:
God Moments: Did That Just Happen
The Desperate Prayer

So the take home message is that for my life and my family's life, food has made a huge difference! I am in awe when I realize what an impact intentional eating (and mindful eating), has had on our lives. I am overcome with emotion when I think about how everything has changed since we started intentional and mindful eating!

Just to recap, in case you missed it. Since I made intentional efforts to eat foods every week that are on the list in this book, the following has happened:

- My mood and stress level has improved profoundly.
- Because I am in a better mood, I make better, more kind choices. (Don't we often act our worst when we are upset, stressed, and hurting.)
- My acne has finally cleared up!
- My allergies and asthma have never been more under control
- My son's anxiety, mood, and behavior has improved tenfold! (Hangry is REAL!)
- In the past, I have gotten severe allergy-related mucus drainage multiple times a year EVERY YEAR. This past fall and spring I did not have this miserable issue for the first time in years!!!
- My energy is off the charts. Recently my friend said, "you are not a morning person or night person; you are an all the time person!" This comment was eye-opening for me as far as how much this way of eating has affected by energy levels.

Okay enough about me, let's move onto other people's real life stories...

First I want to share is a case study published in Child Adolescent Psychiatry and Mental Health. In this case, a 16-year-old teenage boy was diagnosed with mixed mood disorder symptoms with psychotic features. His symptoms, which had been ongoing for a year, were irritability, aggressive behavior, apathy, crying and truancy.

His treatment team discovered that he had a B12 deficiency so they started him on Vitamin B12 supplements. By the second week after giving him B12 supplements, he showed no psychotic features!

I share this as an example of how much nutrients and nutrient deficiencies can impact our health!

The last story I want to share is about a friend. My friend had noticed that he was feeling irritated and upset often. He decided to change his eating. He had been eating fast food everyday for work, but instead of ultra-processed fried foods, he started bringing in things like omega-3-rich walnuts and sautéed vegetables for lunch. He noticed something surprising: he was in a much more cheerful mood! In fact, his mood changes were so noticeable that even his friends started commenting about the change!

Nutrients and Addiction Recovery
Before moving on, I wanted to address addiction recovery in its own section because many of the foods in this book, can aid in addiction recovery. In fact, eating any of these foods promotes overall good health which is beneficial to recovery. However, there are certain foods that are particularly significant when it comes to addiction recovery.

Many people who suffer from addiction have mental, emotional, or physical pain and use these addictive substances to self-medicate. Therefore, feeding the brain foods that improve mood and focus, while providing energy and alleviating some pain, can aid in addictive recovery.

Promoting gut health is also important for people with opiate addictions because opiates can damage the GI organs. Alcohol damages several organs including the liver. The liver is responsible for detoxifying the body. Alcohol addiction can lead to diabetes, liver cirrhosis, heart disease, and malnutrition. All of these conditions are connected to our nutritional health. So, again, nutrition is crucial for anybody who wants to be active in recovery.

****

So, I hope you can see why food is a true gift from God. I think a lot of us have heard of many of these nutrients, and we know that they are beneficial. But when I say these nutrients are crucial, I hope I have convinced you of the magnitude of this statement!

A Little Caveat

One last thing before we get to reason number 2 for this book….I do want you to read this with a grain of salt. Yes! Let's celebrate that these foods are strongly linked to all kinds of benefits and can reduce the risk and improve all kinds of conditions, but there is no guarantee.

I know this personally. When my husband and I decided to try to get pregnant, I started eating foods that promote a healthy pregnancy. Before even becoming pregnant, I omitted foods that could increase the risk of a miscarriage. I still had a miscarriage when I was 3 months pregnant. With my second pregnancy and even more with my third pregnancy, I relaxed a little. I still ate healthy, but in moderation. Both, pregnancies went well. The point is I don't want you to food obsess.

These foods are amazing, and we should try to eat them and enjoy them often. But when you are craving foods on the "less healthy list" and decide to eat them, that is okay too.

Remember Reason number 2 was to provide a quick and easy way to get these nourishing foods on the table everyday.

In my first book, I showed you how I make a month of meals in one day. Talk about easy! You cook once a month and eat healthy everyday!

But now I have a new resource for you! Say you don't want to plan and prep meals each week, but you still want to eat healthy….

And perhaps you don't even want to cook freezer meals every month, but you still want to eat healthy…

Is there another convenient easy way to get healthy meals on the table? Well, I guess you already know what I am going to say…
why yes…yes there is!

You can use "The Nourishing Meal Builder" resources to put together a healthy meal everyday that promotes healing, provides immune supportive and mood boosting ingredients, and reduces the risk or alleviate symptoms of chronic disease, autoimmune diseases, AND improves cognitive function.

Here is How It Works

First pick your base from the Base list or Base cards (provided in chapter 6). Then you pick a protein or two from the Protein List or Protein Cards. Next you pick as many vegetables as you want from the vegetable list or vegetable cards. Now you pick the seasoning and sauces from the list or cards. I grouped seasonings and sauces together so that no matter which combination of sauces you pick on the card/list, they will ALWAYS taste fantastic together (preferences vary, of course)! Finally, you pick from the add-in list/cards and you pick your cooking method from the list provided.

No more digging though recipes or looking into the fridge trying to figure out what to cook! You can combine these lists and cards together and in one minute you have a nourishing and tasty recipe!

Moreover, you can even select and omit cards based on what foods you have available in the house!

Or you can take the cards with you to the grocery store. No more need for grocery lists!

You see, I have always loved to cook, but I found that I didn't have the time or the mental energy to figure out what to eat everyday. Trying to juggle girl scouts, soccer practice, dance class, volunteer meetings, work, cleaning the house, and all the other "mom" duties along with meal prepping and meal planning was just causing too much stress.

The mental load was just too much to bear. This is no longer an issue any more! I was able to reduce my mental load and stress in two ways. One, through making freezer meals, and two, by creating "The Nourishing Meal Builder! I use a combination of both based on my mood and time.

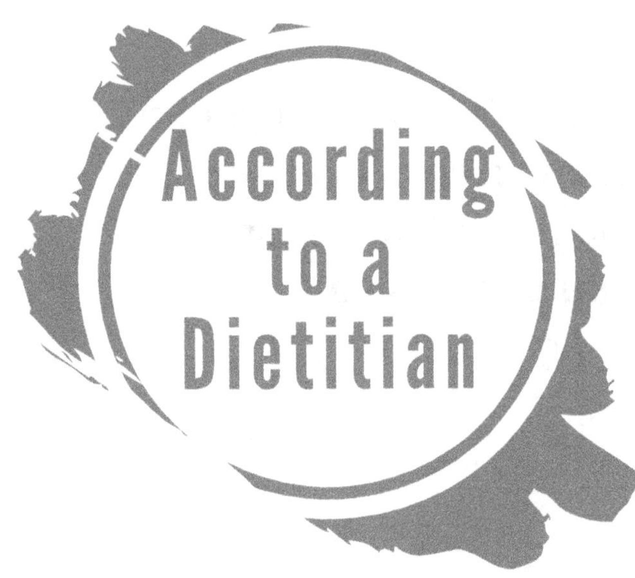

CHAPTER 2
INCORPORATE THESE NUTRIENTS IN YOUR DIET TO

REDUCE THE RISK OR ALLEVIATE THE SYMPTOMS OF THE FOLLOWING CONDITIONS:

- Heat Disease
- Stroke
- Diabetes
- Inflammation
- Rheumatoid Arthritis
- Fibromyalgia
- Distention
- Bloating
- IBS and IBD
- Leaky Gut
- Heartburn
- Migraines
- Diarrhea
- Constipation
- Stomach Pain & Cramps
- Fatigue/Decrease Energy Levels
- Headaches
- GERD
- Gas
- Frequent Colds & Illnesses
- Alzheimer's Disease
- Dementia
- Autoimmune diseases
- Cancer
- Mucus drainage & phlegm
- Allergies
- Brain function like lack of focus and attention
- Memory problems
- Joint Pain
- Hormone imbalance
- Mood disorders like depression, anxiety, stress,
- Acne,
- Insomnia
- Inability to lose weight
- Small Intestine Bacteria Overgrowth
- Crohn's Disease
- Lupus
- Ulteracitive Colitis
- Celiac Disease
- MS
- Parkinsons

Chapter 2:
Nutrients to Incorporate into Your Life

Okay so you can see that food interacts with our body in a profound way. Now it's time to get to the good stuff. As promised earlier, below is a list of nutrients that may reduce the risk or alleviate the symptoms of the following conditions:

Heat Disease, Stroke, Diabetes, Inflammation, Cancer, Rheumatoid Arthritis, Fibromyalgia, Distention, Bloating, IBS, Leaky Gut, Heartburn, Migraines, Diarrhea, Constipation, Stomach Pain and Cramps, Fatigue/Decrease Energy Levels, Headaches, GERD, Gas, Frequent Colds and Illnesses, Autoimmune diseases, mucus drainage and phlegm, Allergies, Memory problems, Joint Pain, Hormone imbalance, Mood disorders like depression, anxiety, and stress, Acne, Insomnia, Inability to lose weight, IBD, Small Intestine Bacteria Overgrowth, Chron's Disease, Lupus, Ulteracitive Colitis, MS, Diabetes, and Parkinson's Disease.

As you go through this nutrient list and later the food list, you will notice that many of these nutrients help with the same condition in multiple ways. For example, leafy greens are a prebiotic. Prebiotics improve gut health, which can help with immune function. Leafy greens are also a source of folate and fiber. Both of these nutrients help with immune function as well!

List of Nutrients and How They Help:

Antioxidants

Reduces oxidative stress and protects your cells from free radicals. See the benefits of specific antioxidants below.

Vitamin A

Alpha-Carotene and Beta-carotene found in fruits and vegetables are a pre-cursor to vitamin A. In other words, the body makes Vitamin A from Beta-carotene.

- Promotes gut health by repairing the gut lining. (Poor gut health, alone, has been linked to many of the medical conditions listed above)
- Antioxidant
- Promotes a healthy immune system
- Has anti-inflammatory properties
- Helps with mood disorders like depression, anxiety, stress
- Has cancer fighting properties
- Reduces risk of heart disease and stroke
- Promotes healthy skin and hair
- Promotes healthy vision
- May improve energy levels/ fatigue
- May reduce cognitive decline and the risk of Alzheimer's and Dementia
- Aids in addiction recovery
- May help with asthma and seasonal allergies

Vitamin E

- Promotes gut health by repairing the gut lining. (Poor gut health, alone, has been linked to many of the medical conditions listed above)
- Antioxidant
- Promotes a healthy immune system
- Has anti-inflammatory properties
- Helps with mood disorders like depression, anxiety, stress
- Reduce the risk of cancer
- Reduce risk of heart disease and stroke
- May improve energy levels/ fatigue
- May reduce cognitive decline and the risk of Alzheimer's and Dementia
- Aids in addiction recovery
- May help with asthma and seasonal allergies

Vitamin C

- Promotes gut health by repairing the gut lining. (Poor gut health, alone, has been linked to many of the medical conditions listed above)
- Antioxidant
- Promotes a healthy immune system
- Has anti-inflammatory properties
- Helps with mood disorders like depression, anxiety, stress
- Reduces the risk of cancer
- Reduces risk of heart disease and stroke
- May improve energy levels/ fatigue
- May reduce cognitive decline and the risk of Alzheimer's and Dementia
- Aids in addiction recovery
- May help with asthma and seasonal allergies

Polyphenols

- Have anti-inflammatory properties
- Antioxidant
- Promote a healthy gut (Remember poor gut health, alone, has been linked to many of the medical conditions listed above)
- Reduce the risk of heart disease and stroke
- Reduce the risk of cancer
- May reduce the risk of Alzheimer's Disease, Dementia
- Helps with mood disorders like depression, anxiety, stress
- Aids in addiction recovery
- May help with asthma and seasonal allergies
- Promotes a healthy immune system

Flavonoids (a polyphenol)

- Prebiotic (good bacteria in the gut feeds on prebiotics)
- Promote gut health by repairing the gut lining. (Remember poor gut health, alone, has been linked to many of the medical conditions listed above)
- Antioxidant
- May reduce the risk of cancer
- Have anti-inflammatory properties
- Reduces the risk of heart disease and stroke
- May reduces cognitive decline and the risk of Alzheimer's Disease, Dementia
- Helps with mood disorders like depression, anxiety, stress
- May help with asthma and seasonal allergies
- Promotes a healthy immune system

Selenium (Some nutrients like Selenium may fall into multiple categories. Selenium has antioxidant properties and is a mineral.)

- May reduce the risk of cancer
- Has anti-inflammatory properties
- Promotes gut health by repairing the gut lining. (Remember poor gut health, alone, has been linked to many of the medical conditions listed above)
- Reduces the risk of heart disease and stroke
- May reduces cognitive decline and the risk of Alzheimer's Disease, Dementia
- Helps with mood disorders like depression, anxiety, stress
- May help with asthma and seasonal allergies
- Promotes a healthy immune system

Glutathione

- Promotes gut health by repairing the gut lining. (Remember poor gut health, alone, has been linked to many of the medical conditions listed above)
- Promotes a healthy immune system
- Has anti-inflammatory properties
- Help with mood disorders like depression, anxiety, stress
- Has cancer fighting properties
- Reduces risk of heart disease and stroke
- May improve energy levels/ fatigue
- May reduce cognitive decline and the risk of Alzheimer's and Dementia
- May help with asthma and seasonal allergies

Quercetin and Kaempferol (Flavonoids)

- Promotes gut health by repairing the gut lining. (Poor gut health, alone, has been linked to many of the medical conditions listed above)
- Immune supportive
- Antioxidant
- Has anti-inflammatory properties
- Helps with mood disorders like depression, anxiety, stress
- Reduce the risk of cancer
- Reduce risk of heart disease and stroke
- May improve energy levels/ fatigue
- May reduce cognitive decline and the risk of Alzheimer's and Dementia
- Aids in addiction recovery
- May reduce seasonal allergy and asthma symptoms
- May help with asthma and seasonal allergies

B vitamins such as Folate/Folic Acid and B12

(B vitamins include: B1: Thiamine; B2: Riboflavin; B3: Niacin; B5: Pantothenic Acid; B6' B7 Biotin; B12, Folic Acid/Folate)
Varying benefits include:

- Helps with mood disorders like depression, anxiety, stress
- May improve energy levels/ fatigue
- Helps your body use energy from food
- Promotes a healthy immune system
- Reduces the risk of cancer
- May improve GI Inflammation (Remember poor gut health, alone, has been linked to many of the medical conditions listed above)
- Aids in addiction recovery
- Supports healthy bones, muscles, and nerves
- Deficiencies in vitamin B6, B12, and folic acid have been linked to increased symptoms of autism.

Minerals

Potassium

- Needed for heart and muscles function
- Helps maintain water and electrolyte balance in your body

Zinc

- Deficiency may increase depression, anxiety, and ADHD symptoms
- Promotes a healthy immune system
- Aids in addiction recovery

Iron

- Promotes healthy immune function
- Deficiency causes anemia and fatigue

Magnesium

- Helps your body use energy from food
- Supports healthy bones, muscles and nerves
- Deficiencies are associated with increased anxiety symptoms, breast cancer, increased risk of heart disease, and increased inflammation
- May help with asthma and seasonal allergies

Calcium

- Important for bone health
- Aids in sleep (Sleep also reduces the risk of these chronic conditions. Isn't it amazing how connected everything it?!?!)

Fiber

- Some fiber is Prebiotic (Good bacteria in the gut feeds on prebiotics; all prebiotics are fiber, but not all fiber is prebiotic)
- Reduce the risk of cancer
- Has anti-inflammatory properties
- Promotes healthy digestion
- Immune supportive

- May reduce joint pain and arthritis inflammation
- Reduces the risk of heart disease and stroke
- Helps you feel full after eating; thus, helps with satiety and weight loss
- Reduces the risk of some cancers
- Help with mood and mood disorders like depression, anxiety, stress
- Protects against diabetes

Other Fat-Soluble Vitamins

Vitamin D

- Promotes gut health by repairing the gut lining. (Remember poor gut health, alone, has been linked to many of the medical conditions listed above)
- May improve mood and help with mood disorders like depression, anxiety, stress
- May improve gut inflammation
- Low levels of Vitamin D have been associated with Autoimmune diseases, skin issues, reduced immune function, increased inflammation, cancer, mood disorders such as depression, stress, anxiety, increased symptoms from ADD and ADHD, Autism, and joint pain and arthritis.
- May help with asthma and seasonal allergies

Vitamin K

- Has anti-inflammatory properties
- Important for Bone health, Heat Disease, and Blood clotting

*If you are taking a blood thinner, you may have to decrease your vitamin K intake

Healthy Fats

Omega-3 Polyunsaturated fat

- May help with joint Pain/arthritis
- Has anti-inflammatory properties
- May improve energy levels/ fatigue
- Helps with mood and mood disorders like depression, anxiety, stress
- Reduces the risk of heart disease
- Improve Gut microbial health and gut inflammation (Remember poor gut health, alone, has been linked to many of the medical conditions listed above!!!)
- Promotes gut health by repairing the gut lining. (Again, remember poor gut health, alone, has been linked to many of the medical conditions listed above)
- May reduce cognitive decline and the risk of Alzheimer's and Dementia
- May improve memory
- Aids in addiction recovery
- May help with asthma and seasonal allergies

Monounsaturated Fat

- Reduces the risk of heart disease
- Promotes a healthy immune system
- May reduce cognitive decline and the risk of Alzheimer's and Dementia

Prebiotics

- Promotes a healthy gut (Good bacteria in the gut feeds on prebiotics, and remember poor gut health, alone, has been linked to many of the medical conditions listed above)
- Promotes a healthy immune system
- May help with asthma and seasonal allergies

Probiotics: Live Good Bacteria Found in Food

- Promotes gut health by repairing the gut lining. (Remember poor gut health, alone, has been linked to many of the medical conditions listed above)
- Boosts immune function
- Has anti-inflammatory properties
- Helps with mood and mood disorders like depression, anxiety, stress
- Reduce the risk of cancer
- Reduce risk of heart disease and stroke
- May improve energy levels/ fatigue
- May reduce cognitive decline and the risk of Alzheimer's and Dementia
- May reduce the risk of some autoimmune diseases
- Aids in addiction recovery
- May helpw with asthma and seasonal allergies

L-glutamine

- Promotes gut health by repairing the gut lining. (Remember poor gut health, alone, has been linked to many of the medical conditions listed above)

L-Thiamine

- Anti-anxiety properties: relaxes or calms the brain without making you drowsy
- May improve mental focus and cognitive performance
- May have immune boosting properties.

Beta Glucan

- Immune supportive
- May help with asthma and seasonal allergies

Lycopene

- May reduce the risk of heart disease and stroke
- May help with asthma and seasonal allergies

Melatonin or Melatonin Precursors (Tryptophan and Serotonin)

- Promotes better sleep at night and relaxation during the day
- Serotonin is a neurotransmitter that makes you feel happy
- Aids in addiction recovery

Mindfulness & Mindful Eating

Okay so this is not a nutrient, but I can't write a book about health without listing mindfulness and mindful eating. The fact of the matter is, mindful eating has have a huge impact on my healthy, mood, and happiness.

Mindfulness & Mindful Eating Benefits

- Promotes gut health; chewing slowly promotes better digestion and decreases stress (Remember poor gut health, alone, has been linked to many of the medical conditions listed above)
- May help with mood and emotions like stress
- May improve energy levels/ fatigue

I have included a chapter on mindfulness & mindful eating at the end of this book.

A Note about these Nutrients

I have not listed every essential nutrient for a couple of reasons. One, you only need trace amounts of many of the nutrients not listed, and we are currently getting plenty of them in the American diet. These are nutrients like Sodium, Chlorine, Phosphorus, and Copper. Plus many of the foods that contain these crucial nutrient listed above also contain these other essential nutrients so if you are eating the foods that contain the nutrients listed above then you are getting enough of the other nutrients.

Some of the nutrients are considered essential nutrients, meaning the body cannot function properly without them. Others listed are not considered essential, but are nutrients that promote health and reduce the risk of chronic diseases and conditions.

I also did not list every function of each nutrient. In other words, these nutrients do even more for your body than what is listed here!!!! In this book, I focused on how these nutrients aid in prevention or treatment of chronic conditions.

Chapter 3:
So What Foods Should I Eat to Get these Nutrients?

Now that we know just how wonderfully beneficial these nutrients are, the next question is 'which foods contain these awesome nutrients?'

Below is a list of food sources of these amazing nutrients:

Fruit

Oranges

- Good source of Vitamin C, fiber, potassium, & folate
- Antioxidant
- Has Anti-inflammatory properties
- Promotes a healthy immune system
- May reduce the risk of cancers
- May improve mood, depression, and stress
- Reduces the risk of heart disease and stroke
- Reduces the of Alzheimer's and Dementia
- May help with asthma and seasonal allergies

Tangerines

- Good source of Vitamin C
- Antioxidant
- Has Anti-inflammatory properties
- Promotes a healthy immune system
- May reduce the risk of cancers
- May improve mood, depression, and stress
- Reduces the risk of heart disease and stroke
- Reduces the risk of Alzheimer's and Dementia

Papaya

- Good source of Vitamin C, fiber, & folate
- Antioxidant
- Has Anti-inflammatory properties
- Promotes a healthy immune system
- May reduce the risk of cancers
- May improve mood, depression, and stress
- Reduces the risk of heart disease and stroke
- Reduce the risk of Alzheimer's and dementia

Grapefruit

- Good source of Vitamin C, fiber, & vitamin A
- Antioxidant
- Has Anti-inflammatory properties
- Promotes a healthy immune system
- May reduce the risk of cancers
- May improve mood, depression, and stress
- Reduces the risk of heart disease and stroke
- Reduces the risk of Alzheimer's and Dementia
- May help with asthma and seasonal allergies

Raspberries

- Good source of fiber and vitamin C
- Polyphenol Antioxidant
- May improve brain function, focus, and attention
- May reduce the risk of Heart disease and stroke
- May reduce the risk of cancer
- Feeds good bacteria
- May reduce the risk of Parkinson's Disease
- May reduce the risk of Alzheimer's and Dementia
- Has Anti-inflammatory properties
- May Increase energy
- Aid in addiction recovery

Mangoes

- Prebiotic (feeds good bacteria and promotes gut health; see the benefits of gut health)
- Good source of Beta-carotene, fiber and vitamin C
- Antioxidant
- Promotes a healthy immune function/immune support
- May reduce depression, stress and enhance mood
- Increase energy
- Promote radiant skin
- May help with Asthma
- Reduce the risk of cancer
- Reduce the risk of heart disease and stroke
- Aid in Digestive health
- Have Anti-inflammatory properties
- May help with Joint pain

Plums

- Polyphenol antioxidant
- May reduce the risk of heart disease
- May reduce the risk of some cancers
- May improve brain function, focus, and attention
- Feeds good bacteria
- May help improve mood, depression, and stress

Apples

- Source of fiber, vitamin C, & Polyphenol antioxidant
- Prebiotic (Feeds good bacteria; see Gut Health Benefits)
- May decrease the risk of heart disease
- May decrease the risk of cancer
- May improve brain function, focus, and attention
- Helps you feel full after eating; thus, helps with satiety and weight loss
- May help with asthma and seasonal allergies

Tart Cherries

- Good source of fiber, vitamin E, & Vitamin A
- Prebiotic (feeds good bacteria and promotes gut health; see gut health benefits)
- Polyphenol antioxidant
- Good source of Melatonin (One of the few food sources of melatonin)
- May help the brain function, focus, and attention
- May reduce the risk of cancer
- May reduce the risk of heart disease and stroke
- May improve mood, depression, stress, and anxiety
- Promotes a healthy immune system
- Aids in sleep
- Aids in relaxation
- May reduce arthritis and joint pain
- May reduce muscle soreness

Cranberries

- Polyphenol Antioxidant
- Fiber-rich
- May improve brain function, focus, and attention
- May improve mood, depression, stress, and anxiety
- May reduce the risk of cancer
- May improve energy levels/fatigue
- Reduce the risk of heart disease and stroke
- May reduce Asthma symptoms
- Reduce the risk of heart disease and stroke
- ·Have Anti-inflammatory properties
- May help with Joint pain
- May reduce the risk of Alzheimer's and Dementia
- May reduce the risk of Parkinson's

Blueberries

- Polyphenol and flavonoid Antioxidants
- Good source of fiber and vitamin C
- Prebiotic (feeds good bacteria and promotes gut health; see gut health benefits)
- May improve brain function, focus, and attention
- May reduce the risk of Alzheimer's and Dementia
- May reduce the risk of Parkinson's
- Have Anti-inflammatory properties
- May improve mood, depression, stress, and anxiety
- May reduce the risk of cancer
- Reduce the risk of heart disease and stroke
- May help with joint pain and arthritis inflammation
- May help with energy
- Provide Immune support
- May reduce Asthma symptoms
- Aid in addiction recovery

Apricots

- Good source of Vitamin A, Vitamin C, & Fiber
- Antioxidant
- May help with gut health by repairing the gut lining. (See benefits of gut microbial health)
- Promotes a healthy immune function
- Have Anti-inflammatory
- Help with mood disorders like depression, anxiety, stress
- Have cancer fighting properties
- Reduce risk of heart disease and stroke
- May improve energy levels/ fatigue
- Helps you feel full after eating; thus, helps with satiety and weight loss

Bananas

- Source of Vitamin B6, Folate, Potassium, Vitamin C, & Fiber
- Antioxidant
- Prebiotic (Feeds good bacteria; see Gut Health Benefits)
- Promotes a healthy immune system
- May decrease the risk of cancer
- Promotes a positive mood, may help with mild depression, stress, and anxiety
- Helps you feel full after eating; thus, helps with satiety and weight loss
- Have Anti-inflammatory properties

- Increases energy
- May improve brain function, focus, and attention
- May reduce the risk of heart disease and stroke
- May help with joint pain and inflammation
- Aid in addiction recovery

Grapes

- Antioxidant
- Good source of Vitamin C
- May help with gut health by repairing the gut lining, reducing GI inflammation, (See benefits of gut microbial health)
- Promotes a healthy immune system
- Have anti-inflammatory properties
- May improve energy levels/fatigue
- Reduce the risk of heart disease and stroke
- May reduce joint pain and arthritis inflammation
- Help you feel full after eating; thus, helps with satiety and weight loss
- Reduces the risk of some cancers
- May help with mood, depression, anxiety, stress
- May help with asthma and seasonal allergies

Blackberries

- A flavonoid and good source of Vitamin C and fiber
- Antioxidant
- May improve immune function/ immune support
- Have anti-inflammatory properties
- Reduce the risk of heart disease and stroke
- May reduce joint pain and arthritis inflammation
- Help you feel full after eating; thus, helps with satiety and weight loss
- Reduces the risk of some cancers
- May help with mood, depression, anxiety, stress
- Promote gut health and improve GI Inflammation (See benefits of a healthy gut!)
- Improve energy
- Promote radiant skin
- Promote brain function, focus, attention
- Aid in addiction recovery
- May reduce the risk of Alzheimer's and Dementia
- May reduce the risk of Parkinson's

Acai Berries

- A good source of fiber
- Antioxidant
- Immune supportive
- Have anti-inflammatory properties
- Reduce the risk of heart disease and stroke
- May reduce joint pain and arthritis inflammation
- Help you feel full after eating; thus, helps with satiety and weight loss
- Reduces the risk of some cancers
- May help with mood, depression, anxiety, stress
- Promote gut health and improve GI Inflammation (See benefits of a healthy gut!)
- Promote brain function, focus, attention, and may help with memory
- Aid in addiction recovery
- May reduce the risk of Alzheimer's and Dementia

Strawberries

- Polyphenol and Flavonoid Antioxidant, Vitamin C
- May improve brain function, focus, and attention
- May reduce the risk of Heart disease and stroke
- May reduce the risk of cancer
- May reduce the risk of Alzheimer's and Dementia
- May reduce the risk of Parkinson's
- Promote a healthy immune system
- Have anti-inflammatory properties
- May improve mood, depression, stress, and anxiety
- Improves energy
- Aid in addiction recovery

Vegetables

Yellow Squash

- Source of Vitamin A, Vitamin C, Folate, fiber, Potassium, and B Vitamins
- Low in Calories, so it adds bulk and fiber to your food without adding many calories so eating it can aid in weight loss
- Antioxidant
- May help with gut health by repairing the gut lining, reducing GI inflammation, (See benefits of gut microbial health)
- Supports a healthy immune system

- Has Anti-inflammatory properties
- May improve energy levels/fatigue
- Reduce the risk of heart disease and stroke
- May help with joint pain and arthritis inflammation
- Reduce the risk of some cancers
- May help with mood, depression, anxiety, stress
- GI Inflammation (See benefits of a healthy gut!)

Zucchini

- Source of Vitamin A, Vitamin C, Vitamin B6 and other B vitamins
- Antioxidant
- Low in Calories, so it adds bulk and fiber to your food without adding many calories so eating it can aid in weight loss
- ·May help with gut health by repairing the gut lining. (See benefits of gut microbial health)
- Promote a healthy immune function
- Has Anti-inflammatory properties
- May help with mood disorders like depression, anxiety, stress
- Reduce the risk of cancer (Cancer fighting)
- Reduce risk of heart disease and stroke
- May improve energy levels/ fatigue

Spaghetti Squash

- Source of Vitamin A, Vitamin C, Folate, fiber, and B Vitamins
- Low in Calories, so it adds bulk and fiber to your food without adding many calories so eating it can aid in weight loss
- Polyphenol Antioxidant
- May help with gut health by repairing the gut lining, reducing GI inflammation, (See benefits of gut microbial health)
- May improve immune function
- Has Anti-inflammatory properties
- May improve energy levels/fatigue
- Reduce the risk of heart disease and stroke
- May help with joint pain and arthritis inflammation
- May reduce the risk of some cancers
- May help with mood, depression, anxiety, stress
- May help with GI Inflammation (See benefits of a healthy gut!)

Kale

- Polyphenol Antioxidant (quercetin)
- Good source of Vitamin A, Vitamin C, Vitamin E, Vitamin K, ALA Omega-3, Fiber, glutathione, Folate, and B vitamins
- Prebiotic (feeds good bacteria and promotes gut health; see gut health benefits)
- May improve brain function, focus, and attention
- May reduce the risk of Alzheimer's and Dementia
- May reduce the risk of Parkinson's
- Supports the immune system
- Has Anti-inflammatory properties
- May improve mood, depression, stress, and anxiety
- May reduce the risk of cancer
- May improve energy levels/fatigue
- Reduce the risk of heart disease and stroke
- May help with joint pain and arthritis inflammation
- Low in Calories, so it adds bulk and fiber to your food without adding many calories so eating it can aid in weight loss
- GI Inflammation (See benefits of a healthy gut!)
- Promotes radiant skin
- May help with Asthma and seasonal allergy symptoms
- Aid in addiction recovery

Corn

- Source of Fiber, Vitamin C, Magnesium, antioxidant, Folate and other B vitamins
- May help with gut health by repairing the gut lining. (See benefits of gut microbial health)
- Supports the immune function
- Has Anti-inflammatory properties
- May improve energy levels/fatigue
- May help with mood disorders like depression, anxiety, stress
- Reduces the risk of cancer
- Reduce the risk of heart disease and stroke
- Promotes healthy digestion
- May reduce joint pain and arthritis inflammation
- Helps with satiety and weight loss

Broccoli

- Prebiotic (feeds good bacteria and promotes gut health; see gut health benefits)
- Good source of Fiber, Vitamin C, Folate, Vitamin K, ALA Omega-3, Polyphenol Antioxidant, iron
- May reduce the risk of Alzheimer's and Dementia
- May improve brain function, focus, and attention
- ·May Improve Immune Function
- Has Anti-inflammatory properties
- May improve mood, depression, stress, and anxiety
- May reduce the risk of cancer
- May improve energy levels/fatigue
- Reduce the risk of heart disease and stroke

- May help with joint pain and arthritis inflammation
- Low in Calories, so it adds bulk and fiber to your food without adding many calories so eating it can aid in weight loss
- Help with GI Inflammation (See benefits of a healthy gut!)

Cabbage

- Good source of Fiber, Vitamin C, Vitamin B6, Folate, Vitamin K, antioxidants
- May help repair gut lining
- Promotes a healthy immune function
- Has Anti-inflammatory properties
- May help with mood disorders like depression, anxiety, stress
- Reduce the risk of cancer (Cancer fighting)
- Reduce risk of heart disease and stroke
- Promotes healthy skin
- May improve energy levels/ fatigue
- Promotes healthy digestion
- May reduce joint pain and arthritis inflammation
- Low in Calories, so it adds bulk and fiber to your food without adding many calories so eating it can aid in weight loss
- Protects against diabetes

Cauliflower

- Antioxidant
- Prebiotic (feeds good bacteria and promotes gut health; see gut health benefits)
- Good source of Fiber, Vitamin C, Folate, and B vitamins, ALA Omega-3
- May improve brain function and reduce the risk of Alzheimer's and Dementia
- Supports immune system
- Has Anti-inflammatory properties
- May improve mood, depression, stress, and anxiety
- May reduce the risk of cancer
- May improve energy levels/fatigue
- Reduce the risk of heart disease and stroke
- May help with joint pain and arthritis inflammation
- Low in Calories, so it adds bulk and fiber to your food without adding many calories so eating it can aid in weight loss
- May help reduce GI Inflammation (See benefits of a healthy gut!)

Turnip Greens and Collard Greens

- Antioxidant
- Prebiotic (feeds good bacteria and promotes gut health; see gut health benefits)
- Good source of Fiber, Vitamin A, Vitamin C, Iron, Folate, and B vitamins
- May improve brain function and reduce the risk of Alzheimer's and Dementia
- May reduce the risk of Parkinson's
- May Improve Immune Function
- Has Anti-inflammatory properties
- May improve mood, depression, stress, and anxiety
- May reduce the risk of cancer
- May improve energy levels/fatigue
- May reduce the risk of heart disease and stroke
- May help with joint pain and arthritis inflammation
- Low in calories, so it adds bulk and fiber to your food without adding many calories so eating it can aid in weight loss
- May reduce GI Inflammation (See benefits of a healthy gut!)
- Aids in addictive recovery

Spinach

- Antioxidant
- Contains Vitamin A, Vitamin C, Vitamin B6, Iron, Fiber, Folate, ALA Omega-3, Calcium
- Low in calories, so it adds bulk and fiber to your food without adding many calories so eating it can aid in weight loss
- May improve brain function and reduce the risk of Alzheimer's and Dementia
- May reduce the risk of Parkinson's
- Supports immune system
- Has Anti-inflammatory properties
- May improve mood, depression, stress, and anxiety
- May reduce the risk of cancer
- May improve energy levels/fatigue
- Reduce the risk of heart disease and stroke
- May help with joint pain and arthritis inflammation
- May reduce GI Inflammation (See benefits of a healthy gut!)
- Promotes radiant skin
- May reduce Asthma symptoms
- Aids in digestion
- Aids in addiction recovery

Green and Black Olives

- Polyphenol Antioxidant
- May improve brain function, focus, and attention
- May reduce the risk of Heart disease and stroke
- May reduce the risk of cancer
- Has Anti-inflammatory properties
- May improve mood, depression, stress, and anxiety

Beets

- Source of folate, Vitamin C, Manganese, Potassium, Fiber
- Has Anti-inflammatory properties
- Promotes a healthy immune system
- May reduce Asthma symptoms
- May improve brain function, focus, attention
- Reduces the risk of cancer
- Reduces the risk of heart disease and stroke
- May help with Joint pain
- Aids in Digestion
- Aids in Weight Management

Asparagus

- Prebiotic (Feeds good bacteria; see Gut Health Benefits)
- Good source of vitamin A, Vitamin C, Vitamin K, Vitamin E, Folate
- Antioxidant
- May improve brain function and reduce the risk of Alzheimer's and Dementia
- May Improve Immune Function
- Has Anti-inflammatory properties
- May improve mood, depression, stress, and anxiety
- May reduce the risk of cancer
- May improve energy levels/fatigue
- Reduce the risk of heart disease and stroke
- May help with joint pain and arthritis inflammation
- Low in calories, so it adds bulk and fiber to your food without adding many calories so eating it can aid in weight loss
- May reduce GI Inflammation (See benefits of a healthy gut!)

Cabbage

- Good source of Fiber, Vitamin A, Vitamin C, Vitamin B6, Folate, Vitamin K
- Antioxidant
- May help repair gut lining
- Promotes a healthy immune function
- Has Anti-inflammatory properties

Carrots

- Prebiotic (feeds good bacteria and promotes a healthy gut; see the benefits of a healthy gut)
- Source of Vitamin A Beta-Carotene Antioxidant, Fiber, Vitamin K
- Promotes a healthy immune system
- Has Anti-inflammatory properties
- Reduces the risk of cancer
- May improve mood, depression, stress and anxiety
- Promotes radiant skin
- May reduce Asthma symptoms
- May improve brain function, focus, attention
- Reduce the risk of heart disease and stroke
- Aids in Digestion
- May help with Joint pain
- Helps with satieity and Weight Management

Onion

- Good source of Fiber, Vitamin C, Vitamin B6,
- Antioxidant
- May help repair gut lining
- Promotes a healthy immune function
- Has Anti-inflammatory properties
- May help with mood disorders like depression, anxiety, stress
- May reduce the risk of cancer

Sweet Potatoes

- Vitamin A, Vitamin B6, Vitamin C
- Antioxidant
- May improve brain function and reduce the risk of Alzheimer's and Dementia
- May Improve Immune Function
- Has Anti-inflammatory properties
- May improve mood, depression, stress, and anxiety
- May reduce the risk of cancer
- Reduce the risk of heart disease and stroke
- May help with joint pain and arthritis inflammation
- May improve energy/fatigue
- May help with weight loss (fiber helps you feel full which can help with weight loss)
- May help wiht GI Inflammation (See benefits of a healthy gut!)

Mushrooms

- Good source of selenium, Vitamin D (exposed to UV light), Iron, Potassium
- Antioxidants
- Has Anti-inflammatory properties
- Promotes a healthy immune system
- May improve energy/fatigue
- May improve mood, depression, stress, and anxiety
- Reduce the risk of heart disease and stroke
- May reduce the risk of Alzheimer's and dementia
- May help with asthma and seasonal allergies

Bell Pepper

- Good source of vitamin C, Vitamin A, Folate, Vitamin B6, Fiber, Vitamin E
- Antioxidant
- May help with gut health by repairing the gut lining. (See benefits of gut microbial health)
- May improve immune function
- Has Anti-inflammatory properties
- May improve energy levels/fatigue
- May help with mood disorders like depression, anxiety, stress
- Reduces the risk of cancer
- Reduces the risk of heart disease and stroke

Brussels Sprouts

- Source of ALA Omega-3 and antioxidants
- Prebiotic (feeds good bacteria, which improves gut health; see the benefits of a healthy gut)
- Contains Vitamin A, Vitamin C, Vitamin K, Vitamin B6, Folate, Fiber
- May improve brain function and reduce the risk of Alzheimer's and Dementia
- May Improve Immune Function
- Has Anti-inflammatory properties
- May improve mood, depression, stress, and anxiety
- May reduce the risk of cancer
- May improve energy levels/fatigue
- Reduce the risk of heart disease and stroke
- May help with joint pain and arthritis inflammation
- Are a filling food; thus, aids in weight loss
- Helps with GI Inflammation (See benefits of a healthy gut!)

Avocado

- Monounsaturated fat: Healthy fat
- Antioxidant
- Good source Vitamin B6, Vitamin C, Fiber, Folate, Vitamin E, Vitamin K, Magnesium, Potassium
- May improve brain function and reduce the risk of Alzheimer's and Dementia
- May Improve Immune Function (Immune Support)
- Has Anti-inflammatory properties
- May improve mood, depression, stress, and anxiety
- May reduce the risk of cancer
- May improve energy/fatigue
- May help with joint pain and arthritis inflammation
- Filling food; thus, aids in weight loss
- Helps with GI Inflammation (See benefits of a healthy gut!)
- Promotes radiant Skin
- May help with Asthma Management
- May reduce the risk of heart disease and stroke
- Promotes healthy digestion
- Aids in addiction recovery

Tomato/ Tomato Juice

- Good source of Vitamin C, Vitamin A, folate, lycopene
- Antioxidant
- May help with gut health by repairing the gut lining. (See benefits of gut microbial health)
- Promotes a healthy immune function
- Has Anti-inflammatory properties

- Help with mood disorders like depression, anxiety, stress
- Reduces the risk of cancer (Cancer fighting)
- Reduces risk of heart disease and stroke
- May improve energy levels/ fatigue
- May help with Asthma symptoms
- May improve brain function and reduce the risk of Alzheimer's and Dementia
- Aids in addiction recovery
- May help with asthma and seasonal allergies

Grains

Oats

- Whole grain
- Prebiotic (feeds good bacteria, promotes healthy gut; see the benefits of a healthy gut)
- Contains B Vitamin, Fiber, Selenium, Tryptophan, Zinc, Magnesium
- Antioxidant
- May improve brain function and reduce the risk of Alzheimer's and Dementia
- Supports Immune Function
- Has Anti-inflammatory properties
- May improve mood, depression, stress, and anxiety
- Reduce the risk of cancer
- May improve energy levels/fatigue
- Reduce the risk of heart disease and stroke

- May help with joint pain and arthritis inflammation
- Helps with satiety and weight loss/weight management
- Helps with GI Inflammation (See benefits of a healthy gut!)
- Helpful for people with diabetes
- Supports Digestion
- Helps with sleep

Whole Wheat

- Whole grain
- Good source of B Vitamins and Fiber,
- May improve brain function and reduce the risk of Alzheimer's and Dementia
- Supports Immune Function
- May improve mood, depression, stress, and anxiety
- Reduces the risk of cancer
- Improves energy levels/fatigue
- Reduces the risk of heart disease and stroke
- Helps with satiety and weight loss
- Helpful for people with diabetes

BuckWheat

- Whole grain (actually a seed)
- Good source of B Vitamins, folate, fiber, magnesium, zinc, calcium, selenium
- May improve brain function and reduce the risk of Alzheimer's and Dementia
- Supports Immune Function
- May improve mood, depression, stress, and anxiety
- Reduces the risk of cancer
- Improves energy levels/fatigue
- Reduces the risk of heart disease and stroke
- Helps with satiety and weight loss
- Helpful for people with diabetes

Quinoa

- Good Source of fiber, folate, zinc, iron, and Manganese
- Prebiotic (feeds gut bacteria and promotes a healthy gut; see benefits of a healthy gut)
- Whole Grain
- Gluten free
- Antioxidant
- Good source of iron
- May improve brain function and reduce the risk of Alzheimer's and Dementia
- Supports Immune Function
- Has Anti-inflammatory properties
- May improve mood, depression, stress, and anxiety
- Reduces the risk of cancer
- Improves energy levels/fatigue
- Aids in addiction recovery

Brown Rice and Wild Rice

- Whole grain
- Gluten free
- Contains B Vitamins and Fiber,
- May improve brain function and reduce the risk of Alzheimer's and Dementia
- Supports Immune Function
- Has Anti-inflammatory properties
- May improve mood, depression, stress, and anxiety
- Reduces the risk of cancer
- Improves energy levels/fatigue
- Reduces the risk of heart disease and stroke
- Helps with joint pain and arthritis inflammation
- Helps with satiety and weight loss
- May help with GI Inflammation (See benefits of a healthy gut!)
- Helpful for people with diabetes
- Aids in addiction recovery

Legumes (Lentils, Chickpeas, Green Peas, Beans)

Legumes (In General)

- Prebiotic (Feeds good bacteria; see Gut Health Benefits)
- Good source of zinc, protein, iron, fiber, folate
- Antioxidant
- Has Anti-inflammatory properties
- Reduce the risk of cancer
- Reduce the risk of heart disease and stroke
- May help with joint pain and arthritis inflammation
- Helps with satiety and weight loss
- May improve GI Inflammation (See benefits of a healthy gut!)
- Aids in addiction recovery
- Promotes a healthy immune system
- May improve energy levels/ fatigue
- May help with mood, depression, anxiety, stress

Fava Beans

- Good Source of Levodopa, fiber, folate, Magnesium, Manganese, Iron, Protein
- Antioxidant
- May slow the progression, or alleviate symptoms of Parkinson's (If you have Parkinson's, please discuss with your doctor; See note below)
- Prebiotic (feeds good bacteria and promotes gut health; see gut health benefits)
- May improve brain function and reduce the risk of Alzheimer's and Dementia
- Supports Immune Function
- Has Anti-inflammatory properties
- May improve mood, depression, stress, and anxiety
- May reduce the risk of cancer
- Reduce the risk of heart disease and stroke
- May help with joint pain and arthritis inflammation
- Aids in addiction recovery
- Helps with satiety and weight loss/weight management
- May improve GI Inflammation (See benefits of a healthy gut!)
- Improves energy levels/ fatigue

A Not on Fava Beans:

Though research is limited, some small studies have shown that Levodopa found in broad beans (also called fava beans) may help with symptoms of Parkinson's disease. But if you have Parkinson's, it is important to talk with your doctor before eating foods in excess that contain Levodopa. You should continue to take medications per your doctors advice as well. Keep in mind, you could over do it if you are taking medications and eating Levodopa rich foods. This excess could cause dyskinesia in Parkinson's patients.

Black Beans

- Source of fiber, folate, zinc, iron, protein
- Antioxidant
- Prebiotic (feeds good bacteria and promotes gut health; see gut health benefits)
- May improve brain function and reduce the risk of Alzheimer's and Dementia
- Supports Immune Function
- Has Anti-inflammatory properties
- May improve mood, depression, stress, and anxiety
- May reduce the risk of cancer
- Reduces the risk of heart disease and stroke
- May help with joint pain and arthritis inflammation
- Aids in addiction recovery
- Helps with satiety and weight loss/weight management
- May improve GI Inflammation (See benefits of a healthy gut!)
- Improves energy levels/ fatigue

Cannellini Beans

- Good source of fiber, Calcium, Potassium
- Prebiotic (feeds good bacteria and promotes gut health; see gut health benefits)
- Improves energy levels/ fatigue
- Supports Immune Function
- May improve mood, depression, stress, and anxiety
- May help with Asthma symptoms
- May help with Brain function, focus, attention
- Reduce the risk of cancer
- Reduce the risk of heart disease and stroke
- Aids Digestion
- Have Anti-inflammatory properties
- May help with Joint pain
- Hepls with satiety and Weight management
- Aids in addiction recovery

Green Peas

- Prebiotic (Feeds good bacteria; see Gut Health Benefits)
- Contains Vitamin A, Vitamin C, Fiber, Folate, Iron, Vitamin K
- Antioxidant
- May help with gut health by repairing the gut lining, reducing GI inflammation, (See benefits of gut microbial health)
- Supports a healthy immune function
- Has Anti-inflammatory properties
- Improve energy levels/fatigue

- Reduce the risk of heart disease and stroke
- May help with joint pain and arthritis inflammation
- Helps with satiety and weight loss/ weight management
- Reduces the risk of some cancers
- May help with mood, depression, anxiety, stress
- May improve brain function, focus, attention

Chickpeas

- Prebiotic (feeds gut bacteria and promotes a healthy gut; see benefits of a healthy gut)
- Good source of protein, fiber, iron, folate, and vitamin B6, Zinc
- Helps with satiety and weight loss
- May improve brain function and reduce the risk of Alzheimer's and Dementia
- Supports a healthy Immune Function
- Have Anti-inflammatory properties
- May improve mood, depression, stress, and anxiety
- May improve energy levels/ fatigue
- May improve brain function, focus, attention
- May help with Joint pain
- Reduce the risk of cancer
- Reduce the risk of heart disease and stroke
- Aid Digestion

- Good source of fiber, iron, Vitamin B6, and Protein
- May improve mood, depression, stress, and anxiety
- May improve energy levels/ fatigue
- Supports a healthy Immune Function
- May help with brain function, focus, attention
- Reduce the risk of cancer
- Reduce the risk of heart disease
- Have Anti-inflammatory properties
- Aid in Digestion
- May help with joint pain
- Helps with satiety and weight loss/weight maintenance

Nuts and Seeds

Walnuts

- Good source of Omega-3 poly unsaturated fat, Folate, Magnesium, fiber, iron, Vitamin B6, manganese, protein, monounsaturated healthy fat, Vitamin E
- Antioxidant
- May improve brain function and reduce the risk of Alzheimer's and Dementia
- May reduce the risk of neurodegenerative diseases like Parkinson's
- Supports a healthy Immune Function
- Has Anti-inflammatory properties
- May improve mood, depression, stress, and anxiety
- May help with asthma and seasonal allergies

- May help with joint pain and arthritis inflammation
- Reduces the risk of cancer
- Reduces the risk of heart disease and stroke
- Promotes healthy gut bacteria, repairing the lining of the gut, and reduce inflammation (See Gut Health Benefits)
- Helps with satiety and weight loss
- Helpful for people with diabetes; improves blood sugar levels
- Improves energy levels/fatigue

Pistachios

- Good source of Folate, Magnesium, fiber, potassium, Vitamin E, Calcium, Vitamin B6, monounsaturated healthy fat, protein
- Antioxidant
- May improve brain function and reduce the risk of Alzheimer's and Dementia
- May reduce the risk of neurodegenerative diseases like Parkinson's
- Supports Immune Function
- Have Anti-inflammatory properties
- May improve mood, depression, stress, and anxiety
- May help with joint pain and arthritis inflammation
- Reduces the risk of cancer
- Reduces the risk of heart disease and stroke
- Promotes healthy gut bacteria, repairing the lining of the gut, and reduce inflammation (See Gut Health Benefits)

- Helps with satiety and weight loss (Low in calories but high in protein)
- Helpful for people with diabetes; improves blood sugar levels
- Improves energy levels and fatigue

Almonds

- Good source of Vitamin E, Protein, fiber, calcium Magnesium, monounsaturated fat: healthy fat
- Antioxidant
- Promote bone health
- May improve brain function, focus, and attention and reduce the risk of Alzheimer's and Dementia
- May reduce the risk of neurodegenerative diseases like Parkinson's
- Supports a healthy immune system
- Have Anti-inflammatory properties
- May improve mood, depression, stress, and anxiety
- May help with joint pain and arthritis inflammation
- Reduces the risk of cancer
- Reduces the risk of heart disease and stroke
- Promotes healthy gut bacteria, repairing the lining of the gut, and reduce inflammation (See Gut Health Benefits)
- Helps with satiety and weight loss
- Helpful for people with diabetes; improves blood sugar level

- Prebiotic (Feeds good bacteria; see Gut Health Benefits)
- May improve energy/fatigue
- Promotes radiant skin

Chia Seed

- Contains Omega-3, Zinc, protein, fiber, calcium
- Antioxidant
- May improve brain function, focus, and attention, and reduce the risk of Alzheimer's and Dementia
- Supports a healthy Immune Function
- Has Anti-inflammatory properties
- May improve mood, depression, stress, and anxiety
- May help with joint pain and arthritis inflammation
- Reduce the risk of cancer
- Reduce the risk of heart disease and stroke
- ·May improve gut health by repairing the lining of the gut in reducing inflammation (See Gut Health Benefits)
- Improve energy/fatigue
- Helps with satiety and weight loss
- Aids in addiction recovery
- May help with asthma and seasonal allergies

- Prebiotic (Feeds good bacteria; see Gut Health Benefits)
- May improve energy/fatigue
- Promotes radiant skin

Flax Seed

- Prebiotic (Feeds good bacteria; see Gut Health Benefits)
- Polyphenol antioxidant
- Source of Omega-3, Vitamin E, protein, fiber, magnesium, monounsaturated fat: healthy fat
- May improve brain function, focus, and attention
- May reduce the risk of Alzheimer's and Dementia
- · Supports a healthy Immune System
- Have Anti-inflammatory properties
- May improve mood, depression, stress, and anxiety
- May help with joint pain and arthritis inflammation
- Reduce the risk of cancer
- Reduce the risk of heart disease and stroke
- May improve energy/fatigue
- Promotes radiant skin
- Helps with satiety and weight loss and weight maintenance
- Aids in addiction recovery
- May help with asthma and seasonal allergies

Sunflower Seeds

- Good source of Vitamin E, Zinc, Selenium, protein, fiber, monounsaturated fat: healthy fat
- Antioxidant
- Supports a healthy Immune System
- Have Anti-inflammatory properties
- May improve mood, depression, stress, and anxiety
- May reduce the risk of cancer
- Reduce the risk of heart disease and stroke
- May help with joint pain and arthritis inflammation
- Improve energy/fatigue
- May help reduce Asthma symptoms
- May improve brain function, focus, and attention
- Helps with satiety and weight loss/ weight maintenance

Hemp Seeds

- Good source of fiber, antioxidants, protein, Omega-3, and monounsaturated fat: healthy fat
- Antioxidants:
- Supports a healthy Immune System
- Have Anti-inflammatory properties
- May improve mood, depression, stress, and anxiety
- May reduce the risk of cancer
- Reduce the risk of heart disease and stroke
- May help with joint pain and arthritis inflammation
- Improve energy/fatigue
- May help reduce Asthma symptoms
- May improve brain function, focus, and attention
- Helps with satiety and weight loss/ weight maintenance

Meat & Meat Alternative

Tuna

- Good source of DHA Omega-3 poly unsaturated fat, Vitamin B6, protein, monounsaturated fat, tryptophan
- Has Anti-inflammatory properties
- May improve brain function and reduce the risk of Alzheimer's and Dementia
- May reduce the risk of cancer
- Supports a healthy immune system
- May improve mood, depression, stress, and anxiety
- Reduces the risk of heart disease and stroke
- May help with joint pain and arthritis inflammation
- May improve gut health by repairing the lining of the gut and reducing inflammation (See benefits of gut health)
- May help with asthma and seasonal allergies

Chicken Broth

- May reduce mucus in the lungs
- Has Immune Boosting properties
- Has anti-inflammatory properties

Salmon

- Good source of DHA Omega-3 poly unsaturated fat, Vitamin B6, Vitamin D, protein, monounsaturated fat
- Has Anti-inflammatory properties
- May improve brain function and reduce the risk of Alzheimer's and Dementia
- May reduce the risk of cancer
- Supports a healthy immune system
- May improve mood, depression, stress, and anxiety
- Reduces the risk of heart disease and stroke
- May help with joint pain and arthritis inflammation
- May improve gut health by repairing the lining of the gut and reducing inflammation (See benefits of gut health)
- May aid in addition recovery
- May help with asthma and seasonal allergies

Turkey

- Good source of protein, Zinc, Vitamin B6, Selenium, tryptophan, B vitamins
- May reduce the risk of Alzheimer's and dementia
- May improve brain function, focus, and attention
- Promotes a healthy immune system
- A lean meat that promotes satiety and aids in weight loss
- Aids in addiction recovery

Chicken (not fried)

- Good source of Protein, Zinc, Vitamin B6, Selenium, tryptophan
- Helps with satiety and weight loss (weight loss can improve inflammation which helps with a host of problems and conditions including gut health and joint pain; Do you see how they all indirectly relate to each other?)
- May improve brain function and reduce the risk of Alzheimer's and Dementia
- Supports a healthy Immune System
- Helpful for people with diabetes; improves blood sugar level

Fish (In General)

- Good source of protein, vitamin D,
- May improve brain function and reduce the risk of Alzheimer's and Dementia
- May improve mood, depression, stress, and anxiety
- May help with joint pain and arthritis inflammation
- Reduces the risk of heart disease and stroke

Caged-Free Omega-3 Eggs

- Good source of Omega-3, Vitamin D, Folate, Protein
- May improve brain function and reduce the risk of Alzheimer's and Dementia
- Supports a healthy Immune System
- Has Anti-inflammatory properties
- May improve mood, depression, stress, and anxiety
- Reduce the risk of cancer
- May improve energy levels/fatigue
- May help with joint pain and arthritis inflammation
- May improve GI Inflammation (See benefits of a healthy gut!)
- May help with asthma and seasonal allergies

Nutritional Yeast

- A complete protein
- Contains antioxidants, vitamin B12, and Beta Glucan
- May improve brain function and reduce the risk of Alzheimer's and Dementia
- Supports a healthy Immune System
- Has Anti-inflammatory properties
- May improve mood, depression, stress, and anxiety
- Reduce the risk of cancer
- May improve energy levels/fatigue
- May help with joint pain and arthritis inflammation
- May improve GI Inflammation (See benefits of a healthy gut!)
- May help with asthma and seasonal allergies

Spices

Thyme

- Polyphenol antioxidant
- May reduce the risk of heart disease and stoke
- May reduce the risk of some cancers
- May improve brain function, focus and attention
- May improve mood, depression, stress, and anxiety

Turmeric

- May help repair the gut lining
- Has Anti-inflammatory properties
- Enhances anti-bodies and immune cells and promotes a healthy immune system
- May reduce the risk of cancer/ Cancer Fighting
- May improve mood, depression, stress, and anxiety
- May improve brain function, focus, attention
- Reduce the risk of heart disease and stroke
- May help with joint pain/Arthritis
- May reduce the risk of Alzheimer's disease and dementia

(Eat Turmeric with black pepper to get the most benefits)

Rosemary

- Polyphenol antioxidant
- May reduce the risk of heart disease
- May reduce the risk of some cancers
- May improve brain function, focus, and attention
- May help improve mood, depression, and stress

Cinnamon

- Antioxidant
- Good source of manganese, Calcium. Fiber, iron
- Has Anti-inflammatory properties
- Promotes a healthy immune system
- ·Has Anti-bacterial properties
- ·May reduce the risk of some cancers
- Helps with satiety and weight loss
- May improve mood, depression, stress, and anxiety
- May improve brain function, focus, and attention
- May help with joint Pain
- Aids in addiction recovery

Ginger

- Helps restore the cleansing wave
- Has Anti-inflammatory properties
- Polyphenol antioxidant
- May improve brain function, focus, and attention
- Promotes a healthy immune system
- Reduces the risk of heart disease and stroke
- May reduce the risk of some cancers
- May help with joint and muscle pain
- May reduce the risk pf Alzheimer's and Demetia
- May have antimicrobial properties

Sage

- Polyphenol antioxidant
- May reduce the risk of heart disease
- May reduce the risk of some cancers
- May improve brain function, focus, and attention
- May help improve mood, depression, and stress

Garlic

- Prebiotic (Feeds good bacteria; see Gut Health Benefits)
- Source of Vitamin C, Vitamin B6, Manganese, Selenium,
- Promotes a healthy immune system
- Has Anti-inflammatory properties
- May improve mood, depression, stress
- Reduces the risk of cancer
- Anti-viral aspects

Horseradish

- May help with seasonal allergy symptoms
- May help with cold and bronchitis symptoms

Honey

- May help soothe a sore throat and coughing

Cayenne Pepper

- May slightly boost your metabolism for a short period of time after eating it.

Cilantro

- Good source of Vitamin K, Carotenoids, flavonoid
- Antioxidant
- Possible Antimicrobial/antifungal properties
- Has Anti-inflammatory properties
- May improve brain function, focus, and attention
- May reduce the risk of heart disease
- May reduce the risk of some cancers
- May help with joint Pain

Fermented and Probiotic-Rich Foods

Probiotics have a variety of benefits. Yet each probiotic is unique and can impact the body in a combination of different ways. The key is to eat a variety of probiotic-rich foods so that you will get a a variety of positive benefits.

Probiotics:

- Have Anti-inflammatory properties
- Promote a healthy immune function
- Reduces stress-induced brain disorders
- Helps with the cleansing wave
- Improves mood and may reduce depression and stress
- Aids in addiction recovery

- Sauerkraut
- Kimchi
- Fermented Pickles
- Miso
- Kefir
- Tempeh
- Kombucha
- Greek Yogurt

Other

Dark Chocolate

- Polyphenol Antioxidant
- Source of Serotonin (the neurotransmitter that makes you feel happy)
- Promotes a healthy immune system
- May improve brain function, focus, attention, and memory
- Promotes a healthy gut
- Has anti-inflammatory properties
- May reduce the risk of heart disease and stroke
- May reduce the risk of cancer
- May reduce the risk of Alzheimer's and Dementia
- May improve mood, depression, stress, and anxiety (anti-depressant)
- May help with a persistent cough

Black Tea, Green Tea, & Mathca

- Polyphenol antioxidant
- May reduce the risk of heart disease and stoke
- May reduce the risk of some cancers
- May improve brain function, focus and attention, and reduce brain fof
- May improve mood, depression, stress, and anxiety
- Has Anti-inflammatory properties
- Decreases the stress hormone, cortisol (possibly because the physical act of mindfully drinking tea is relaxing. When drinking tea, you notice the smells, the warmth of the cup, and the calming heat from the steam)
- Contains L-theanine (L-Theanine relaxes the brain without making you drowsy); Black tea contains more
- May decrease the risk of Alzheimer's and Dementia
- Promote a healthy immune system
- Slightly increases metabolism
- May increase brain performance o cognitive tests
- May help with focus and improve motor abilities (particularly Matcha)

Coffee (Plain)

- Polyphenol antioxidant
- May reduce the risk of heart disease
- May reduce the risk of some cancers
- May improve brain function, focus, and attention
- May decrease the risk of Parkinson's disease
- Has anti-inflammatory properties
- Reduces the risk of Type 2 diabetes

- May have anti-anxiety properties (due to the L-thiamine)
- Decreases the stress hormone, cortisol (possibly because the physical act of mindfully drinking tea is relaxing. When drinking tea, you notice the smells, the warmth of the cup, and the calming heat from the steam)
- Contains L-thiamine (L-Thiamin relaxes the brain without making you drowsy

Extra Virgin Olive Oil

- Antioxidant
- Monounsaturated Fat: Healthy fat
- May improve brain function, focus, and attention
- May reduce the risk of Heart disease and stroke
- May reduce the risk of Alzheimer's and Dementia
- May improve mood, depression, stress, and anxiety
- May reduce the risk of cancer
- May reduce the risk of type 2 diabetes

A Note About Oil

Different oils have different positive characteristics. Olive Oil, almond oil, and avocado oil are a great source of monounsaturated fats. Coconut oil is a good source of MCT (medium-chain tryglycerides) oil. Research suggest that MCT oils are metabolized differently and are not stored as fat. MCT oil may even slightly increase metabolism.

Some oils have a beneficial omega-3/omega-6 ratio. Omega-3 and Omega-6 are important for the body; however, the ratio between these two polyunsaturated fats is also very important. Here in the United States, we are getting more omega-6 compared to omega-3. In other words, we are getting too much omega-6 and not enough omega-3s. We should aim for at max a 4:1 omega-6 to omega-3 ratio. In the U.S, the ratio is anywhere from 12:1 to 25:1!!!!! These high omega-6 ratios promote inflammation.

Flax Seed Oil has a 1:4 omega-6 to omega-3 ratio!!!

Final Thoughts

Just by looking at the huge collections of foods on this list, I think it is easy to see that there is not one certain food that is a super food. In fact, optimal health is all about variety. It is not healthy to eat just one thing. Variety seems to hold true among oils too. Based on the data, the Blue Zone, and the Mediterranean diet, I think Extra Virgin Olive Oil should be an oil we use, and use frequently; however, there are benefits to changing up your oils as well.

Foods that Have a Negative Impact on How we Feel, Think, and Function

We have established that food can nourish the mind, body, and soul, but sometimes we eat food for other valid reasons. Sometimes we eat food that may not provide the best nourishment but provide something else. Sometimes we eat food because it brings back a happy memory, or we eat food just because it taste good. (Nourishing or not, I hope we are always eating foods that bring us joy).

It is okay to eat these less nourishing foods occasionally, but when we eat these foods in excess, they can have a negative impact on how we feel, think, and function. So listen to your body and only eat these foods sparingly.

When I started listening to my body, and watching my children's response to food, I realized we felt best when we ate the powerhouse foods 90% of the time.

Foods that can have a Negative Impact on how we Feel, Think, and Function

Refined Sugar and Simple Carbohydrates

Refined sugar and simple carbohydrates promote the growth of "bad" bacteria in the gut; may increase the risk for chronic conditions including Alzheimer's, Dementia, and other brain dysfunctions; decrease immunity; increase inflammation; increase mood disorders like depression, anxiety, and stress; exasperate symptoms of ADHD and Autism; and may have a negative impact on addiction recovery.

Fried Foods

Fried foods promote inflammation which as we have seen earlier can cause a host of problems from poor gut health to pain joint pain. Fried foods may increase the risk of Alzheimer's disease, Dementia, Cancer, and more.

While some alcohol may have some benefits, too much alcohol can cause gut bacteria imbalance, which can snowball into a host of problems (Se gut bacteria health benefits)

Too much beer may increase the risk of Alzheimer's and decrease brain function

The MIND diet has been shown to reduce the risk of heart disease, Alzheimer's, dementia, and other brain dysfunctions, stroke; and more. The MIND diet recommends limiting butter and margarine, which contain saturated fats and trans fat (margarine).

Trans fats could increase the risk of gut imbalance, Alzheimer's, dementia, brain fog, as well as reduce brain function

Limiting vegetable oils could help with gut health (See benefits of gut health list)

Red Meats and Smoked Meats

Too much can increase the risk of cognitive decline, dementia, Alzheimer's, and some cancer; and increase inflammation. (Remember, inflammation can increase the risk of a multitude of conditions.

Milk Chocolate

Milk chocolate may Increase inflammation, and remember, inflammation can increase the risk of a multitude of condition.

Ultra Processed Foods

Limiting processed foods promotes gut balance; reduces the risk of Alzheimer's, dementia, cancer, and inflammation; and improves symptoms of ADHD. Heavily processed, low-fiber foods may reduce brain and immune function and contribute to depression, stress, and poor moods.

Not all "processed" foods are bad. Processing simply means altering a food. Pre-cut vegetables are considered processed because they were cut up (ie altered). However heavily processed foods are the foods you want to limit. When reading the labels on food boxes look for short ingredients lists with simple food listed. Look for whole foods like whole grains, vegetables, nuts, or fruit as the first ingredient on carbohydrate/starchy foods like crackers. Look for foods that have no added sugar or trans fat.

Heavily processed foods include pastries, sausage, salami, bologna, hot dogs, fruit snacks, candy, and some cereals.

Decrease Stress

Okay so this isn't food, but stress can have just as much of an impact, if not more, than food. Stress feeds bad bacteria in the gut, increases inflammation, and suppresses the immune system. Reducing stress may also help with weight loss. So follow the mindful exercises listed in this book and eat foods that have been shown to help with stress.

Food Sensitivities: Temporarily Eliminating Foods

Food sensitivities and intolerances, can contribute to poor gut health. Inversely, poor gut health can increase food sensitivities. Changing your diet can greatly improve your gut health and many symptoms and conditions, but if you are still having problems even after incorporating a healthier diet and following your doctor's medical treatment; then, you may want to try an elimination diet to determine if you have any food sensitivities or food intolerances.

Among people with food sensitivities, some have always had them, while others can become sensitive to a food by eating one food too often. Sometimes, after you have given your body a break from these food sensitivities, you can add the foods back into your diet as part of a VARIED diet. Variety is key so that we do not overeat them again. Others will find that they will have to continue eliminating a food to continue reaping the health benefits and control symptoms.

Gluten is an example of a food Americans could be eating too often, which may be one reason some are becoming sensitive to gluten. In the American diet, we are not getting much variety when it comes to grains. We eat pasta, sandwiches, wraps, pizza, and buns…all made from wheat! So perhaps we should aim for a variety of whole grains instead of only whole wheat. So, for one meal perhaps we could eat whole wheat pasta; then the next meal we could eat brown rice, quinoa, or oats.

Usually you can eliminate the foods you are sensitive to while simultaneously eating foods that improve your gut health. Once you have healed your gut, many people can add those foods back into their diet. Remember though, variety is key.

The most common food sensitivities and intolerances are:

- Gluten
- Dairy
- Soy
- Yeast
- Corn
- Eggs
- Nuts
- Histamine
- FODMAPs
- Nightshade Vegetables
- Cruciferous Vegetables

Although science is somewhat conflicting, other possible intolerances that may exasperate ADHD are artificial colors, especially red and yellow, and food additives such as aspartame and MSG.

Fortunately, eating a whole foods diet will decrease the amount of additives and colors consumed

No one food cures all, but by eating a combination of the Whole Foods listed in this book as well as eating less of the heavily processed foods listed as well, you might just be able to:

- Improve gut bacteria balance
- Decrease leaky gut
- Decrease inflammation
- Decrease Asthma Symptoms
- Decrease the risk of heart disease and stroke
- Lose weight
- Reduce the risk of type 2 diabetes
- Improve ADHD symptoms
- Reduce the risk of cancer
- Improve arthritis symptoms
- Increase good cholesterol (HDL)
- Reduce the risk of dementia and Alzheimer's
- Decrease blood pressure
- Improve mood, depression, and anxiety
- Decrease waist adipose fat
- Improve sleep
- Reduce the risk of liver disease
- Reduce the risk of kidney disease
- Reduce the prevalence of headaches
- Improve energy/fatigue
- ·Reduce the risk of cataracts
- Improve acne
- Decrease food allergies
- Improve menopause symptoms

- Improve IBS, Crohn's and Ulcerative Colitis symptoms
- Decrease GERD
- Possibly reduce Parkinson's disease symptoms
- Improve brain function, focus and attention

MEAL PLAN CHECKLIST

BY LACY NGO, MS, RDN AT MINDFULNESS IN FAITH AND FOOD

A HEALTHY DIET ...	NOTES
☐ Mostly plant-based	
☐ Whole grains: 2-3X/day Alternate whole grains to reduce the likelihood of developing a food sensitivity	
☐ Vegetables: Every meal	
☐ Leafy greens: 1x/day	
☐ Nuts: 5X/week	
☐ Beans/Legumes: 4X/Week	
☐ Poultry: 2X/week	
☐ Fish (Salmon): 2x/week	
☐ Fruit: Everyday	
☐ Berries: 2x/week	

MEAL PLAN CHECKLIST

BY LACY NGO, MS, RDN AT MINDFULNESS IN FAITH AND FOOD

A HEALTHY DIET ...	NOTES

☐ Probiotics : 4-5X/week
(yogurt and cultured foods)

EAT LESS OFTEN

- Refined Sugar
- Added Sugar
- Fried Foods
- Red Meat
- Smoked Meats
- Beer
- Heavily Processed Foods (ex: boxed pastries, hotdogs, bologna, luncheon meats (nitate & nitrite free are better choices), boxed foods with long ingredients lists)

Chapter 5:
How to Build a Meal

Below are the simple steps to building your nourishing meals everyday!

Step 1: Pick your base from the Base list or Base cards (provided in chapter 6).

Step 2: Pick a protein or two from the Protein List or Protein Cards.

Step 3: Pick as many vegetables as you want from the vegetable list or vegetable cards.

Step 4: Pick the seasoning and sauces from one of the Seasoning and Sauces blocks or cards.

 I grouped seasonings and sauces together so that no matter which combination of sauces you pick on the card/list, they will ALWAYS taste fantastic together (preferences vary, of course)! If you desire a more "soupy" or stew-type meal, add more broth and sauces (ex: tomato sauce). If you want a creamier sauce, add the cream cheese, yogurt, or cream soups. For a sandwich, you may want to use less "soupy" ingredients. Seasoning and oils work great together for sautéed vegetables and proteins.

Step 5: Pick a Healthy Addition and/or an occasional cheese if desired.

Step 6: Pick a cooking method from one block or card.

When choosing which brand of seasoning and sauces to use, follow the "Is It Healthy?" chart on the following page. This chart is a helpful reference for choosing packaged snacks as well.

IS IT HEALTHY?

Label Reading Checklist

- Minimal Refined Grains

- A whole food is listed as the first ingredient

- Minimal Added Sugar (No added sugar is best!).

- Simple Ingredients List

- No trans fats

- Contains Beneficial Nutrients (Vitamins, Minerals, Fiber, Antioxidants, Omega 3s, Probiotics, etc)

THE MEAL BUILDER

CHOOSE FROM EACH BLOCK TO
BUILD A MEAL

BASE (CHOOSE 1)

- Oats
- Chickpea Pasta
- Zoodles
- Brown rice
- Palmini
- Black Bean Pasta
- Quinoa
- Whole Grain Pasta
- Cauliflower rice/mashed
- Lentil Pasta
- Whole Grain Pizza crust

- Whole Grain Wraps to make wraps, pizza, tacos, or quesadillas (I like Ole' Xtreme High Fiber)
- Cauliflower pizza crust
- Cauliflower Knochi
- Whole Grain Bread, Sub rolls, buns, English muffins, etc (I like Dave's bread)
- Soba Noodles
- Spring Roll Wrap

- Lettuce Leaves as a Wrap
- Lettuce, Kale, Spinach for a salad
- Cauliflower or Broccoli Tots (I like Green Giants)
- Baked Chips made with whole grains, flaxseed, black beans, or quinoa (Find The Healthiest Chips & Crackers on our blog)
- Crackers made from whole grain, flaxseed, chia seeds, etc)
- Kasha
- Spaghetti squash

PROTEIN (CHOOSE 1)

- Salmon Fillet
- Canned Salmon or Salmon Packets
- Eggs
- Grilled Fish
- Bird'seye Steam Fresh Protein Blends
- Canned Chickpeas
- Canned Tuna or Tuna Packets/Pouches

- Nuts and Seeds (Like almonds, walnuts, Pistaccios, pumpkin seeds, chia seeds, flaxseed, hemp seed, etc.)
- Beans, canned or frozen (any variety: Cannanelli, Kidney, Black Eyed, Black, etc.)
- Grilled Chicken

- Ground Chicken
- Ground Turkey
- Frozen Veggie Burgers (I like Amy's California Veggie)
- No nitrate/nitrite added Turkey Slices
- No Nitrate/nitrite added chicken sausage (I like Applegate)

THE MEAL BUILDER

CHOOSE FROM EACH BLOCK TO
BUILD A MEAL

VEGETABLE (CHOOSE 3 OR MORE)

- Zucchini
- Broccoli
- Corn
- Onion
- Kimchi (Il like Mother In Law Brand)
- Celery
- Sauerkraut (I like Farmhouse Culture Brand)
- Tomato
- Cucumber
- Kale
- Spinach
- Asparagus
- Cherry tomatoes
- Green beans
- Peas
- Sun Dried Tomatoes
- Jar of Capers
- Roasted Red Pepper
- Carrots
- Slaw Packs (Broccoli, Cabbage, Kale, etc)
- Cabbage
- Cauliflower
- Squash (Any variety)
- Brussels Sprouts
- Frozen Vegetable Mixes
- Beans (Any Variety)
- Peppers (Any Variety)
- Avocados
- Sweet Potatoes
- Mushrooms
- Artichokes
- Fermented Pickles
- Salsa
- Pico Del Gallo

SUPER ADD-INS (OPTIONAL)

- Flaxseeds
- Hemp Seeds
- Chia Seeds

CHEESES (OPTIONAL)

- Parmesan
- Mozzarella
- Cheddar
- Goat
- Ricotta
- Nutritional Yeast (Cheese substitute)

THE MEAL BUILDER

SEASONING AND SAUCE
COMBINATIONS
CHOOSE 2 OR MORE FROM 1 BLOCK

ASIAN INSPIRED

- Teriyaki Sauce (Primal Kitchen) or Soy Sauce + choices below:
  - Garlic
  - Sesame Oil
  - Salt
  - Black Pepper
  - Honey + Ketchup (I like Primal Kitchen Brand)
  - Siracha Sauce
  - Mirin
  - For creamy sauce: Cream Cheese, yogurt; or a can of cream soup
  - Asian Vinaigrette
  - Chicken/Vegetable Broth

CURRY

- Tomato sauce + Honey + Seasonings below:
  - Coriander
  - Cumin
  - Turmeric and Black Pepper
  - Garlic
  - For creamy sauce: Cream Cheese, yogurt (add after cooking); or a can of cream soup
  - Ginger
  - Cayenne Pepper
  - Mustard

DRESSINGS AND VINAGARETTES

- Honey + Vinegar
- Balsamic or Cider Vinegar
- Black Pepper
- Chicken/Vegetable broth
- Onion Powder Mix
- Extra Virgin Olive Oil
- White Pepper
- Italian Dressing (I like Primal Kitchen)
- For creamy sauce: Cream Cheese, yogurt (add after cooking); or a can of cream soup

THE MEAL BUILDER

SEASONING AND SAUSE
COMBINATIONS
CHOOSE 2 OR MORE FROM 1 BLOCK

ITALIAN

- Montreal Seasoning
- Tomato Sauce (I like Primal Kitchen)
- Italian Seasoning
- Parsley
- Oregano
- Garlic
- Black Pepper
- Salt
- Honey
- Basil
- Sage
- Tomato Soup Can
- For creamy sauce: Cream Cheese, yogurt (add after cooking); or a can of cream soup)
- White Pepper
- Extra Virgin Olive Oil

BBQ

- Montreal Seasoning
- BBQ Sauce (I like Primal kitchen)
- White Pepper
- Turmeric and Black Pepper
- Garlic
- Worcestershire Sauce

CHILI

- Montreal Seasoning
- Chili Seasoning
- Chicken Broth
- Cream Cheese (For a Creamy Sauce)
- Tomato Sauce (I like Muir Glen)
- Salt
- Yogurt (Add after cooking to preserve live bacteria)
- White Pepper, Black Pepper, or Cayenne Pepper
- Garlic
- Worcestershire Sauce

THE MEAL BUILDER

SEASONING AND SAUSE
COMBINATIONS
CHOOSE 2 OR MORE FROM 1 BLOCK

MARINATE INSPIRED

- Italian Dressing/Vinigarette
- White wine sauce
- Garlic
- Caper's
- Lemon juice
- Parsley
- Chicken Broth
- Vegetable Broth
- Black Pepper
- Salt
- Cider/Balsamic Vinegar
- Extra Virgin Olive Oil

KICKIN' "SAUSAGE"

- Fennel Seeds
- Garlic
- Paprika
- Black Pepper
- Salt
- White Pepper
- BBQ Sauce
- Worcestershire
- For creamy sauce: Cream Cheese, yogurt (add after cooking); or a can of cream soup

SOUTHWEST INSPIRED

- Chipotle Adobe Sauce
- Chicken Broth/ Vegetable Broth
- Taco Seasoning (I like Simply Organic)
- Garlic
- Paprika
- Salt
- Lime Juice
- Lemon Juice
- For creamy sauce: Cream Cheese, yogurt (add after cooking); sour cream, or a can of cream soup
- Tomato Sauce
- Extra Virgin Olive Oil
- Avocado Oil
- Cilantro
- White Pepper
- Cayenne Pepper
- Sriracha Sauce
- Cumin

THE MEAL BUILDER

SEASONING AND SAUSE
COMBINATIONS
CHOOSE 2 OR MORE FROM 1 BLOCK

GET CREATIVE

- Hot sauce
- Montreal Seasoning
- White wine
- garlic
- salt
- pepper
- Chicken/Vegetable broth
- onion soup mix
- Ranch packets
- Worcestershire
- Paprika
- BBQ Sauce
- White Pepper
- Turmeric and Black Pepper
- For creamy sauce: Cream Cheese, yogurt (add after cooking); or sour cream, a can of cream soup
- Extra Virgin Olive Oil
- Salad Dressings made with less sugar and simple ingredients (I like Primal Kitchen)
- Everything but the Bagel Seasoning

PESTO

Choose all on the list, mix in a food processor, Saute' with ingredients from other cards

- Basil
- Leafy Green
- Pine Nuts or other nuts
- Parmesan Cheese
- Garlic
- Olive Oil
- Black Pepper
- Salt

THE MEAL BUILDER

ALFREDO

Use the Ingredients Below to Make a Healthy Alfredo or simply use Primal Kitchen's Alfredo Sauce

- Parmesan
- Garlic
- Salt
- Black Pepper
- Cream Cheese
- Vegetable Broth
- Milk (I like 1 % Omega-3 Milk

SIGNATURE

Mix all the ingredients below to make a Signature Sauce

- Horseradish
- Avocado or Olive Oil Mayo (I like Primal Kitchen)
- Lemon Juice
- BBQ Sauce (Primal Kitchen)
- Honey
- Siracha Sauce

THE MEAL BUILDER

SEASONING AND SAUSE
COMBINATIONS
CHOOSE 2 OR MORE FROM 1 BLOCK

KEEP IT SIMPLE

A Note on Sauces: Choosing healthy condiments, sauces, and dressings can be overwhelming. You want your sauces and condiments to provide nourishment, and yet sometimes you just don't want to make a sauce from scratch. This is why I love the Primal Kitchen Brand. These dressings, condiments, and sauces have no sugar added and use simple whole ingredients. So when I want to keep things simple, I just pick a base, pick my vegetables, pick a protein, and add a Primal Kitchen Sauce or dressing. Bam! My recipe is done!

- **Pick a Primal Kitchen Sauce or dressing, done**

THE MEAL BUILDER

CHOOSE A COOKING METHOD (1 OR MORE)

Saute'	**Bake** *Perfect for mixed and layered casseroles
Slow Cooker	**Pressure Cooker**

THE MEAL BUILDER

CHOOSE A COOKING METHOD (1 OR MORE)

SANDWICH, WRAP, LETTUCE WRAP

DIP WITH CHIPS/ CRACKERS

SALAD

"MEAT"BALL/ PATTY

*Just add egg or flaxseed and water to chosen ingredients and form a ball or patty; bake or sauté

CHOOSE A COOKING METHOD (1 OR MORE)

EGG MUFFIN CUP

Add eggs and ingredients of your choice to a muffin cup and bake

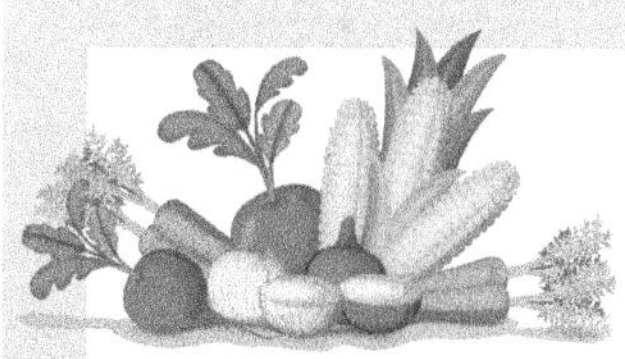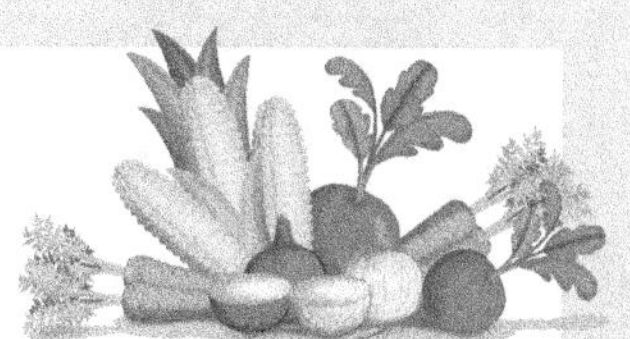

The Meal Builder Cards

For the Mind, Body, & Spirit

Developed by Lacy Ngo, MS, RDN

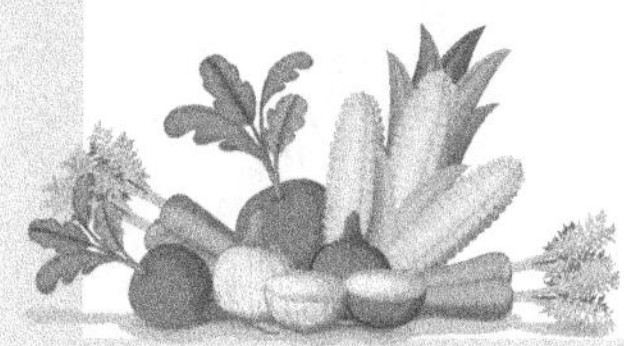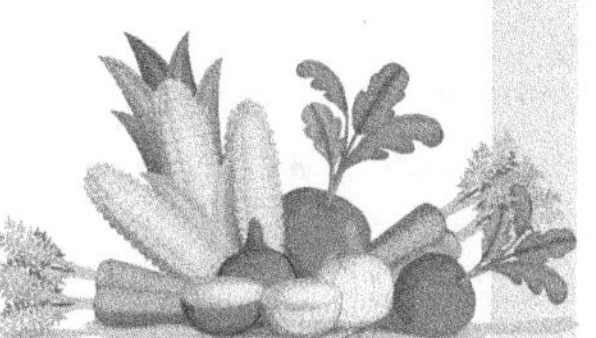

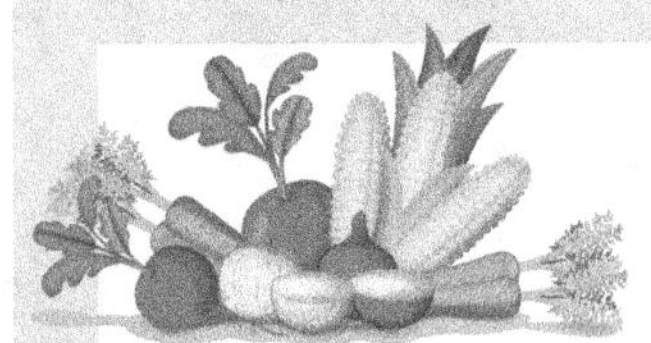 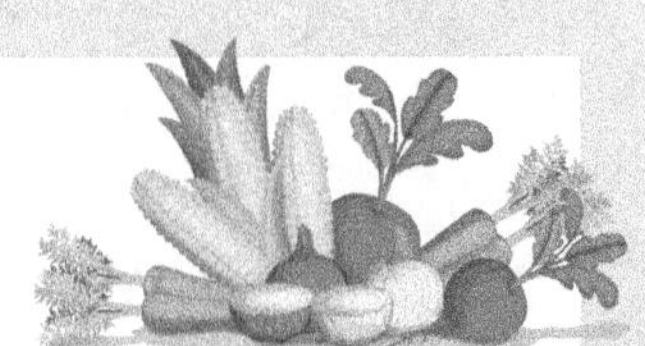

The
Meal Builder
Cards

For the Mind, Body, & Spirit

Developed by Lacy Ngo, MS, RDN

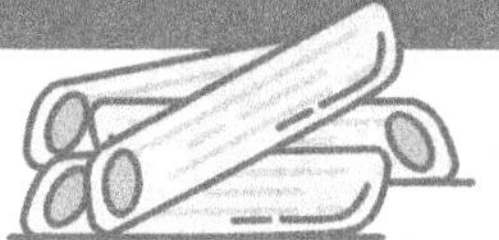 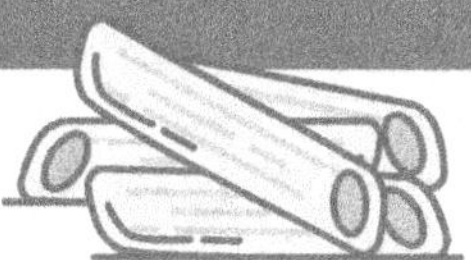

Base (Choose 1)

Oats

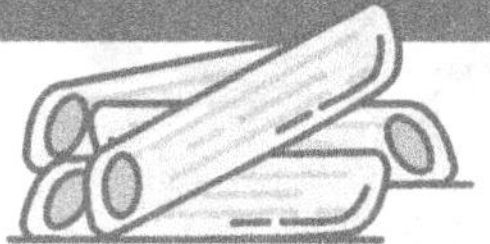 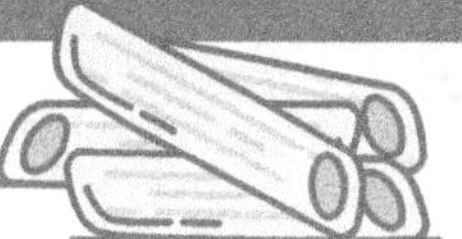

Base (Choose 1)

Chickpea Pasta

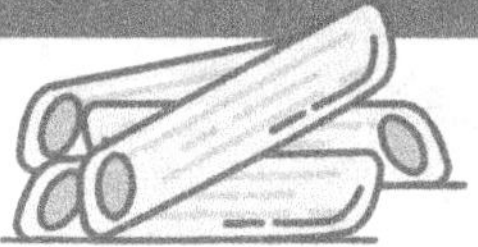 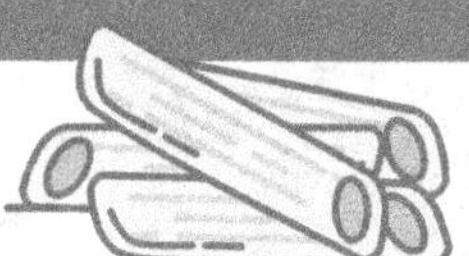

Base (Choose 1)

Zoodles

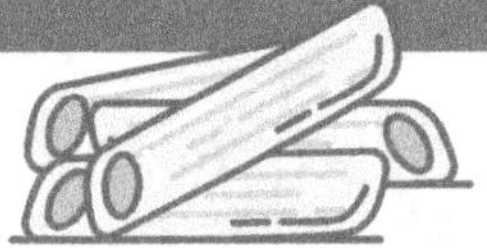 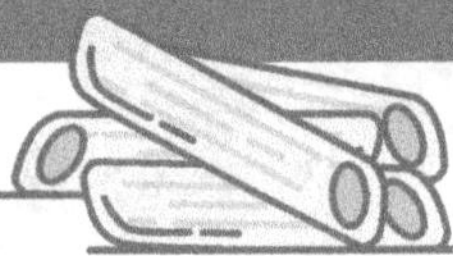

Base (Choose 1)

Brown Rice

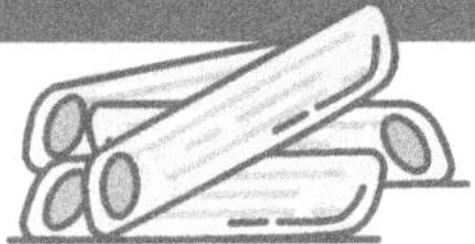 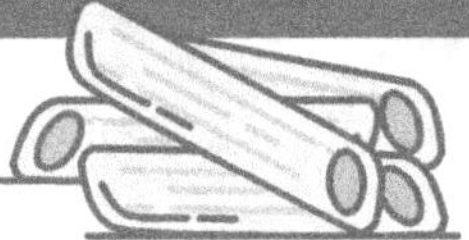

Base (Choose 1)

Palmini

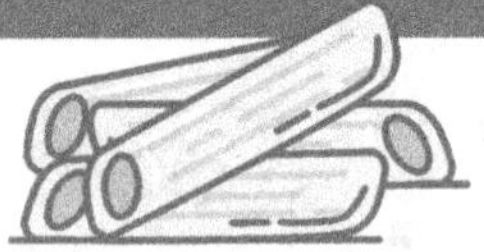 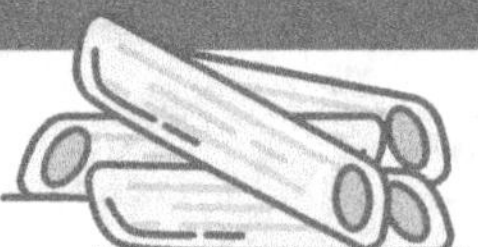

Base (Choose 1)

Black Bean Pasta

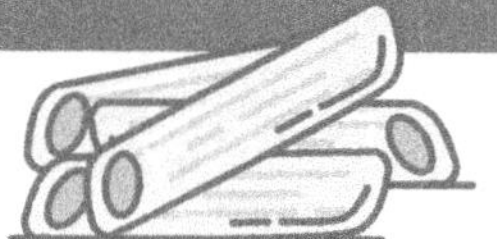 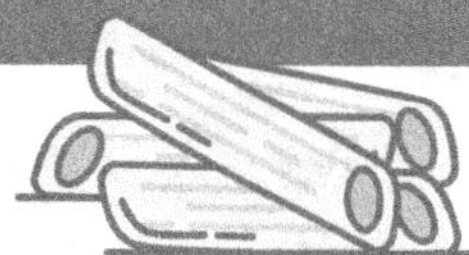

Base (Choose 1)

Quinoa

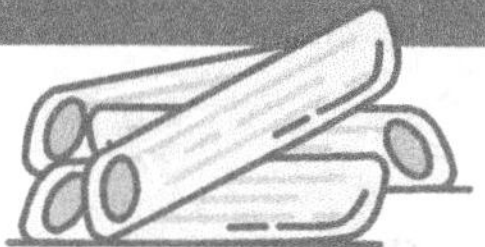 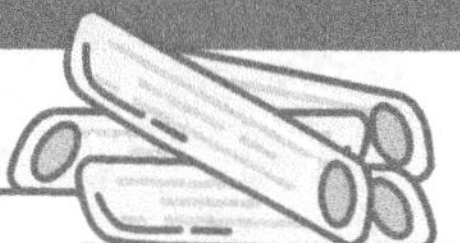

Base (Choose 1)

Whole Grain Pasta

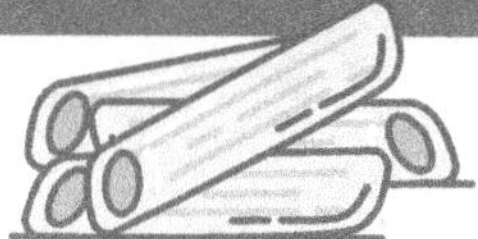 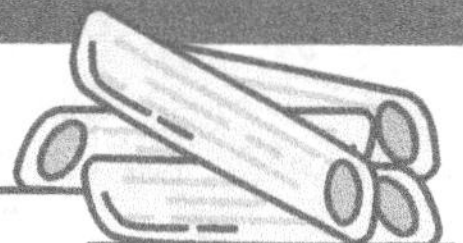

Base (Choose 1)

Cauliflower Rice/Mashed

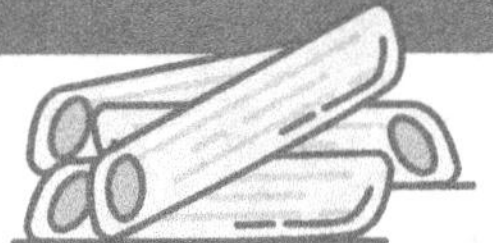 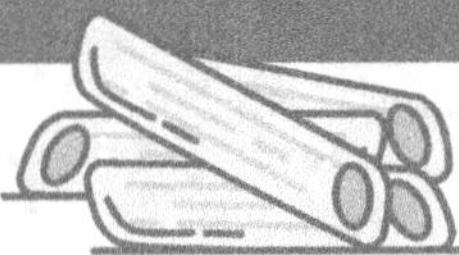

Base (Choose 1)

Lentil Pasta

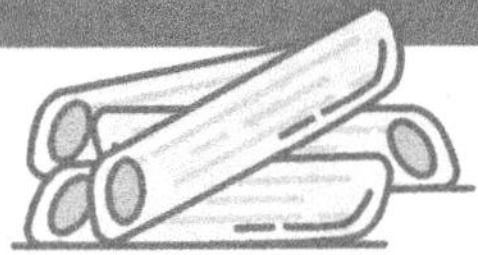 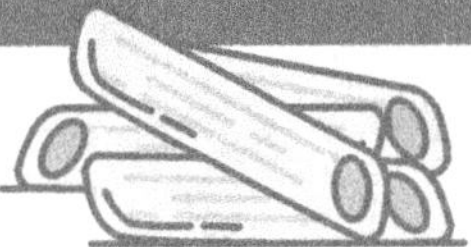

Base (Choose 1)

Whole Grain Pizza Crust

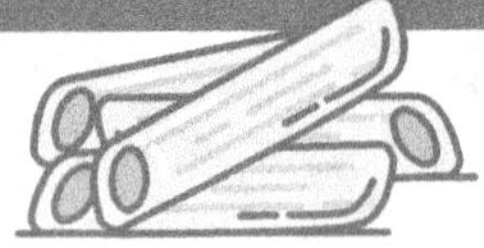 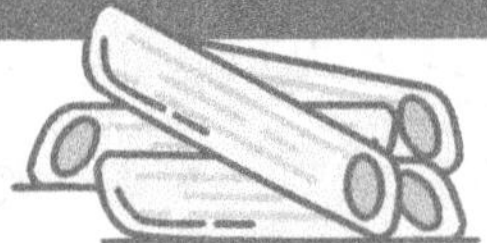

Base (Choose 1)

Whole Grain Wraps to make wraps, pizza, tacos, or quesadillas (I like Ole' Xtreme High Fiber)

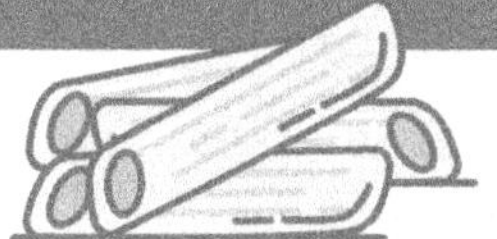 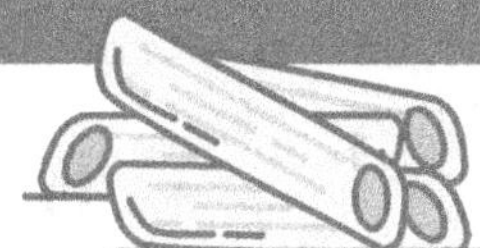

Base (Choose 1)

Cauliflower Pizza Crust

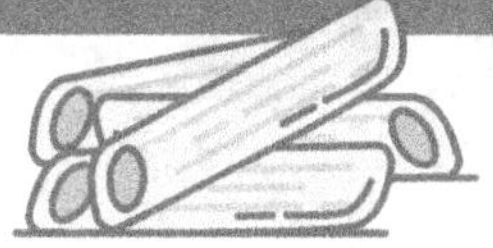 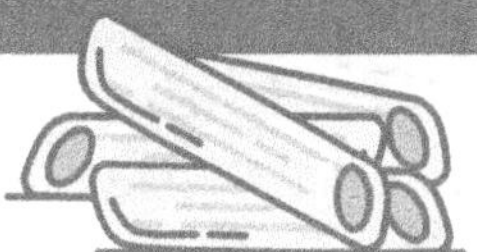

Base (Choose 1)

Cauliflower Knochi

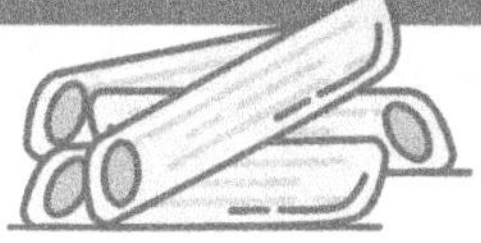 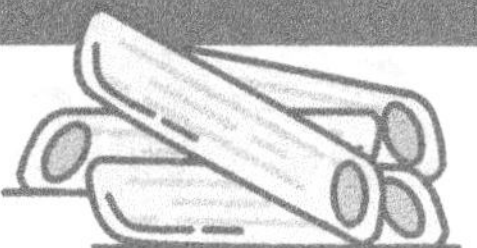

Base (Choose 1)

**Whole Grain Bread,
Sub rolls, buns,
English muffins, etc.
(I like Dave's bread)**

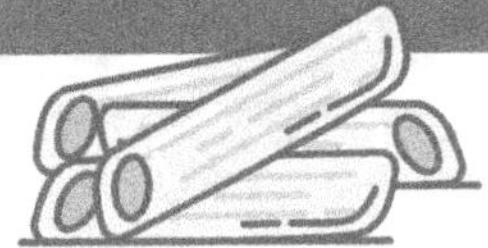 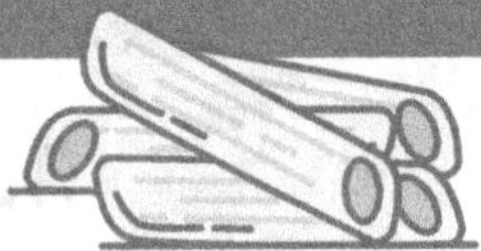

Base (Choose 1)

Lettuce Leaves as a Wrap

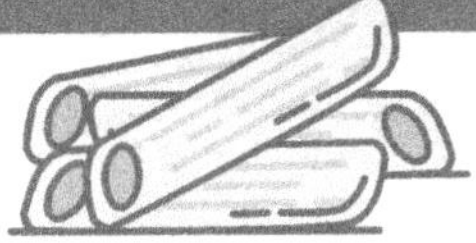 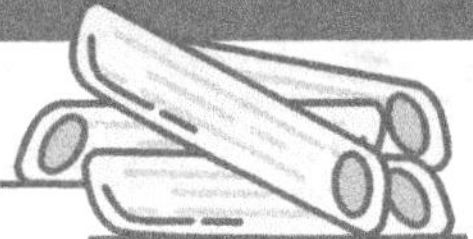

Base (Choose 1)

Lettuce, Kale, Spinach Bed as a Salad

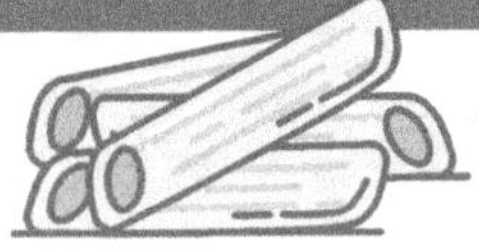 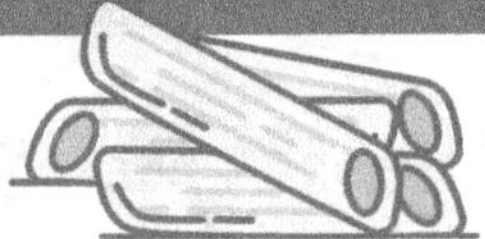

Base (Choose 1)

Cauliflower or Broccoli Tots (I like Green Giants)

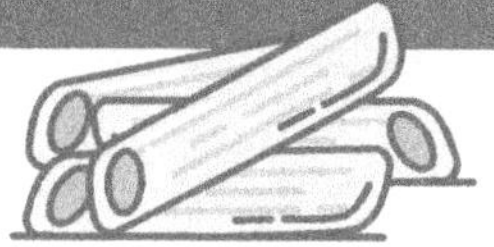 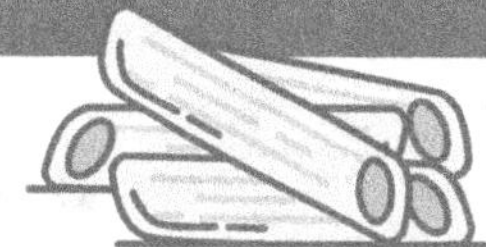

Base (Choose 1)

Baked Chips made with whole grains, flaxseed, black beans, or quinoa

(See our Blog for Heathiest Chips & Crackers list**)**

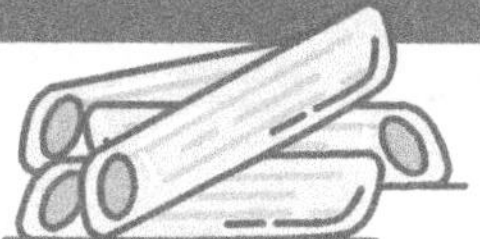 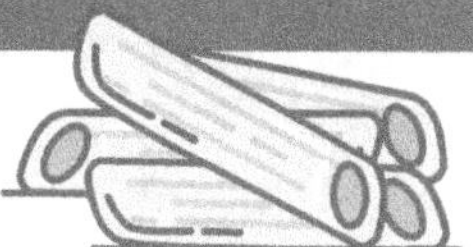

Base (Choose 1)

Crackers made from whole grain, flaxseed, chia seeds, etc)

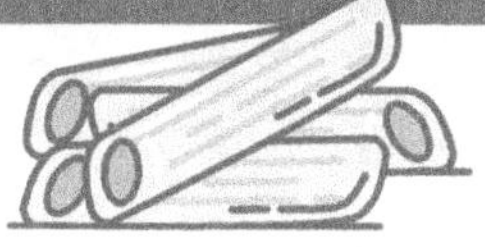 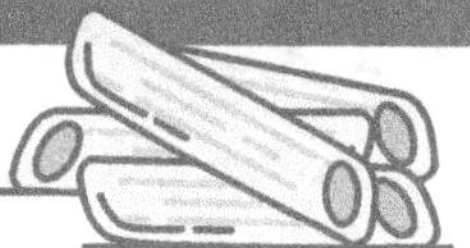

Base (Choose 1)

Soba Noodles

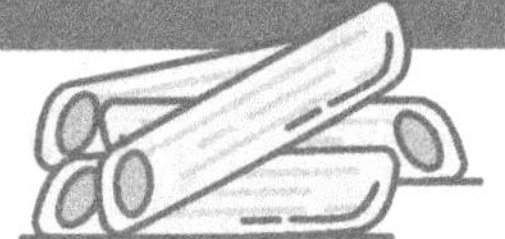 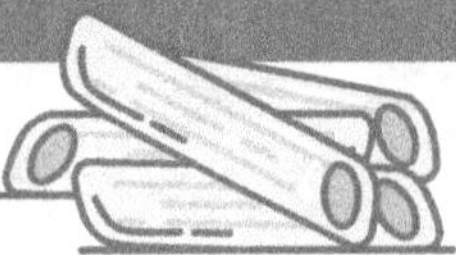

Base (Choose 1)

Kasha

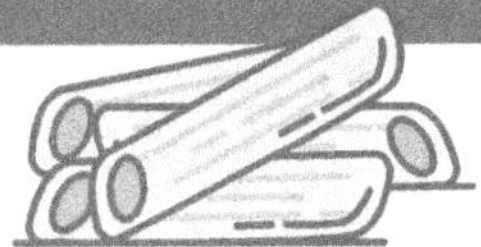 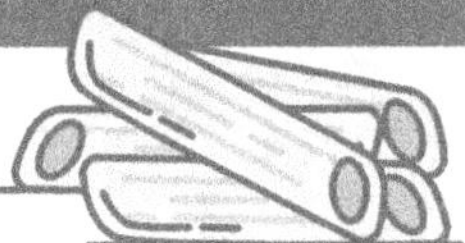

Base (Choose 1)

Spring Roll Wraps

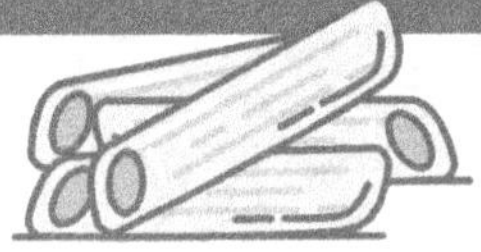 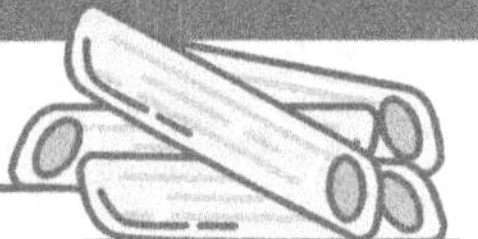

Base (Choose 1)

Spaghetti Squash

 **Protein (Choose 1 or more if Plant-Based)** 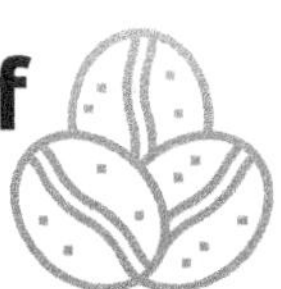

Soy Beans

 **Protein (Choose 1 or more if Plant-Based)** 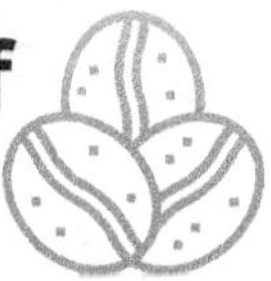

Salmon Fillet

 **Protein (Choose 1 or more if Plant-Based)** 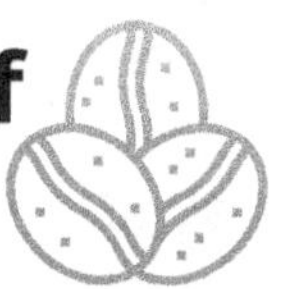

Canned Salmon or Salmon Packets

Protein (Choose 1 or more if Plant-Based)

Eggs

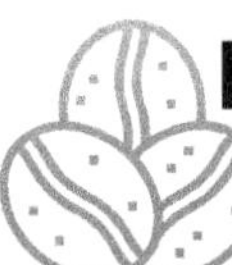 

Protein (Choose 1 or more if Plant-Based)

Grilled Fish

 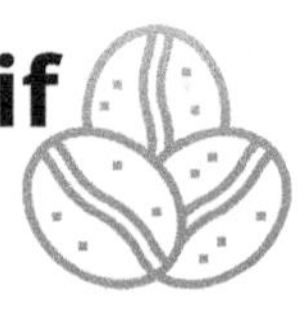

Protein (Choose 1 or more if Plant-Based)

Plant Based Protein Mixes like Bird'seye Steam Fresh Protein Blends

 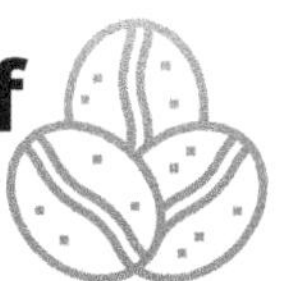

Protein (Choose 1 or more if Plant-Based)

Canned Chickpeas

 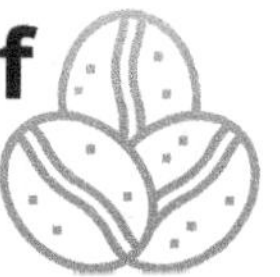

Protein (Choose 1 or more if Plant-Based)

Nuts and Seeds (Like almonds walnuts, Pistaccios, pumpkin seeds, chia seeds, flaxseed, hemp seed, etc.)

Protein (Choose 1 or more is Plant-Based)

Canned Tuna or Tuna Packets/Pouches

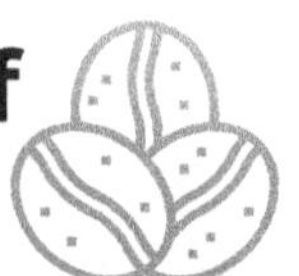

Protein (Choose 1 or more if Plant-Based)

Grilled Chicken

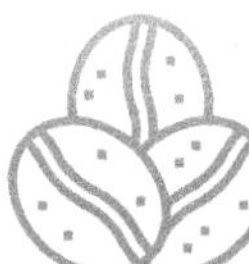

Protein (Choose 1 or more if Plant-Based)

Beans, canned or frozen (any variety: Cannanelli, Kidney, Black Eyed, Black, etc.)

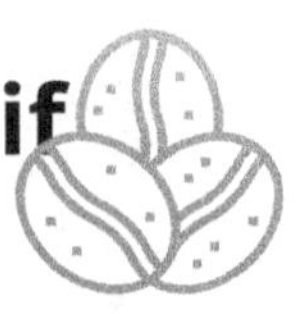

Protein (Choose 1 or more if Plant-Based)

Ground Chicken

 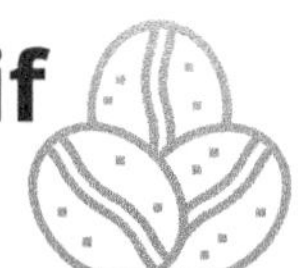

Protein (Choose 1 or more if Plant-Based)

Grilled Turkey

Protein (Choose 1 or more if Plant-Based)

Turkey Slices (No nitrite/nitrate added)

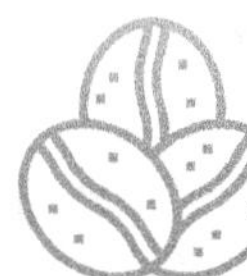 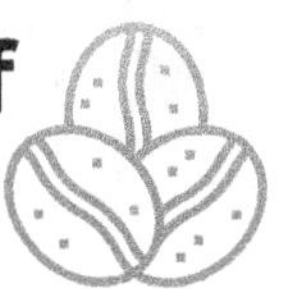

Protein (Choose 1 or more if Plant-Based)

No Nitrate/nitrite added chicken sausage

(I like Applegate)

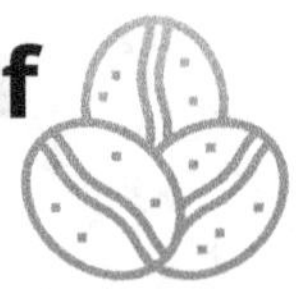

Protein (Choose 1 or more if Plant-Based)

Frozen Veggie Burgers

(I like Amy's California Veggie)

Protein (Choose 1 or more if Plant-Based)

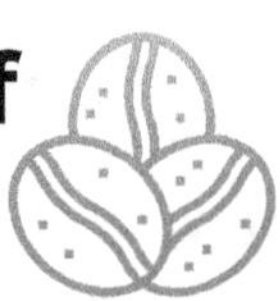

Protein (Choose 1 or more if Plant-Based)

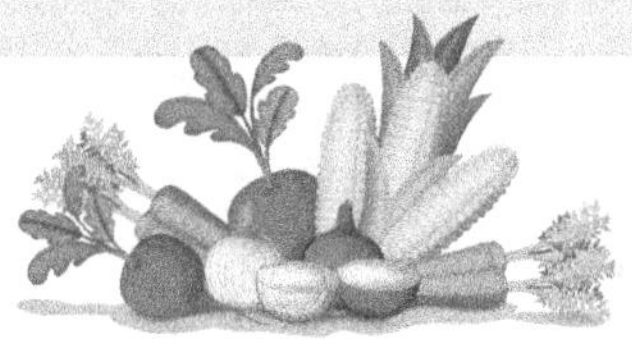 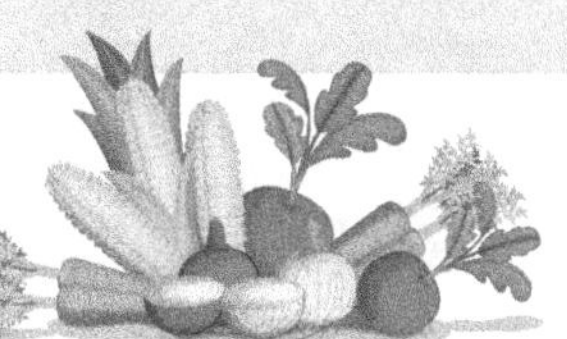

**Vegetables
(Choose 3 or More)**

Zucchini

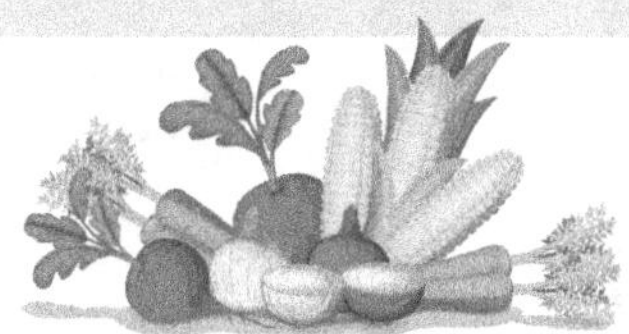 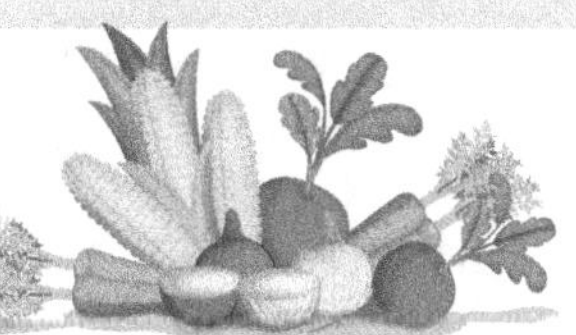

**Vegetables
(Choose 3 or More)**

Broccoli

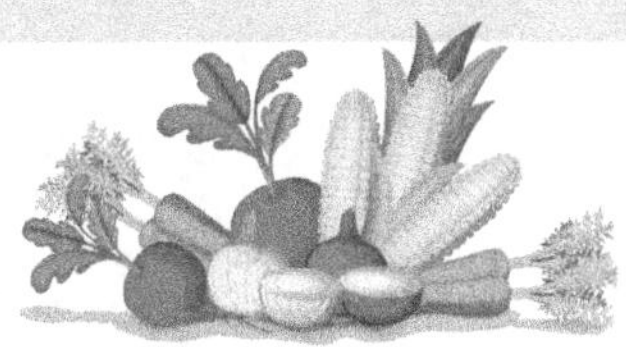 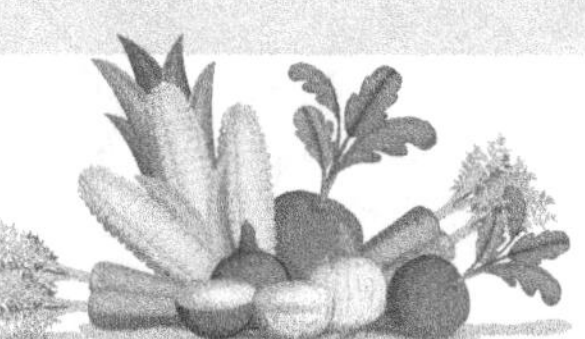

**Vegetables
(Choose 3 or More)**

Corn

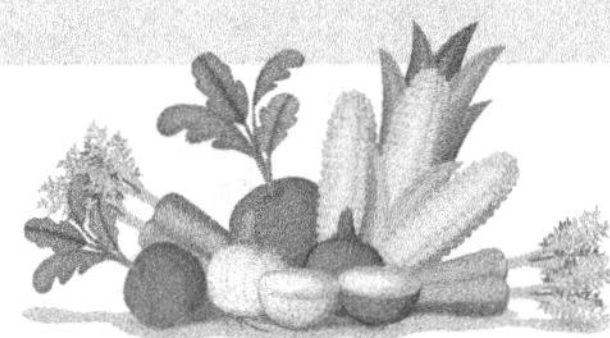 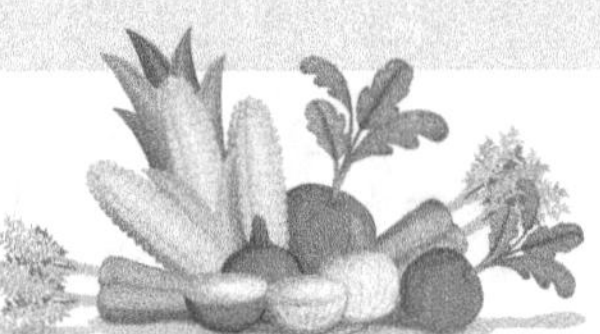

**Vegetables
(Choose 3 or More)**

Onion

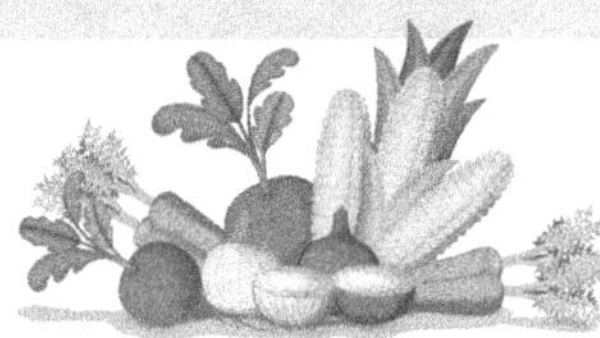 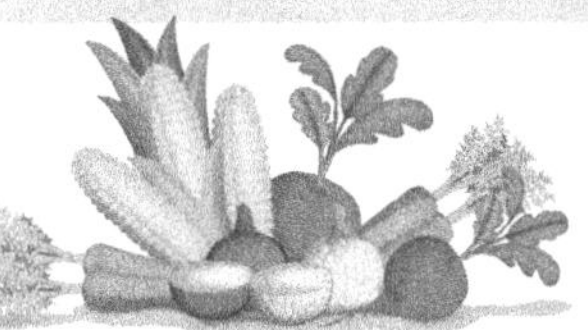

**Vegetables
(Choose 3 or More)**

Kimchi (I like Mother In Law Brand)

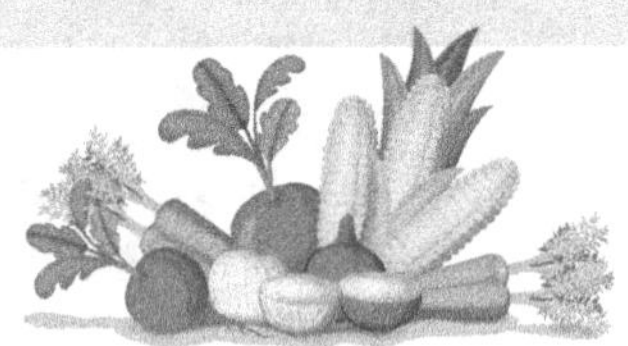 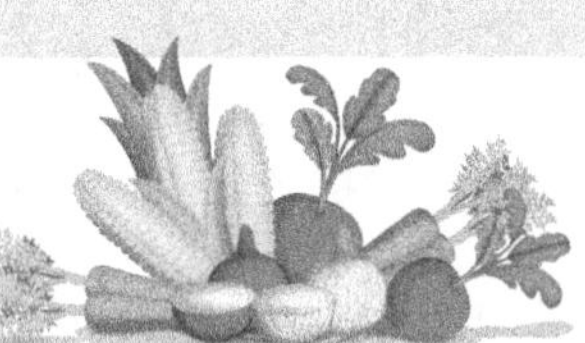

**Vegetables
(Choose 3 or More)**

Celery

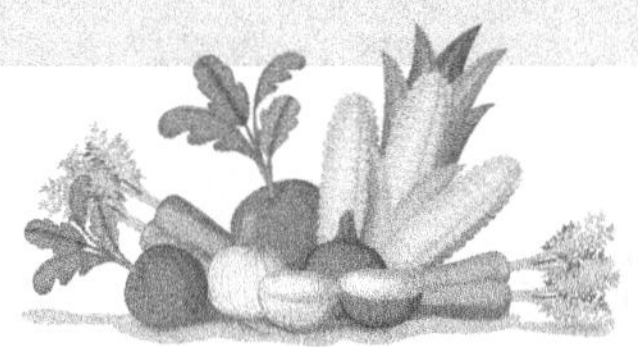 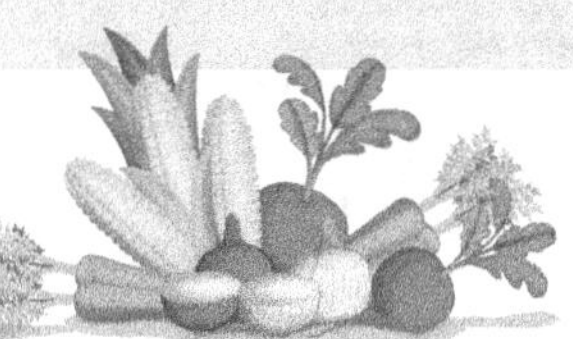

Vegetables
(Choose 3 or More)

Tomato

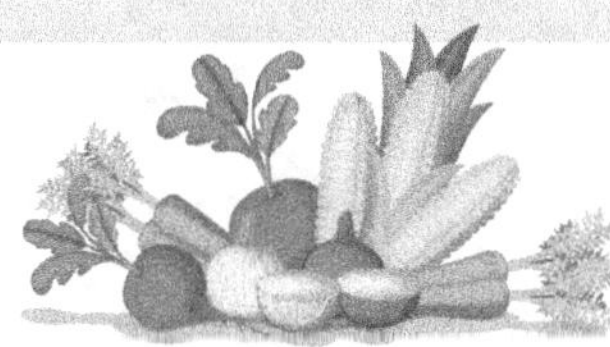 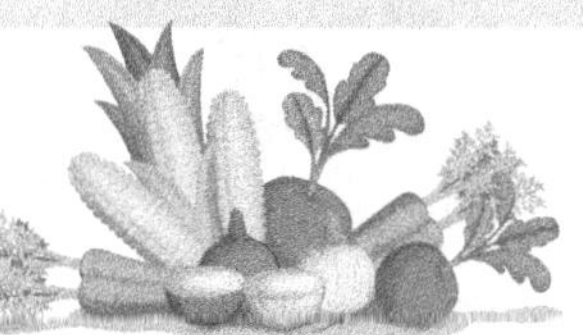

Vegetables
(Choose 3 or More)

Sauerkraut (I like Farmhouse Culture Brand)

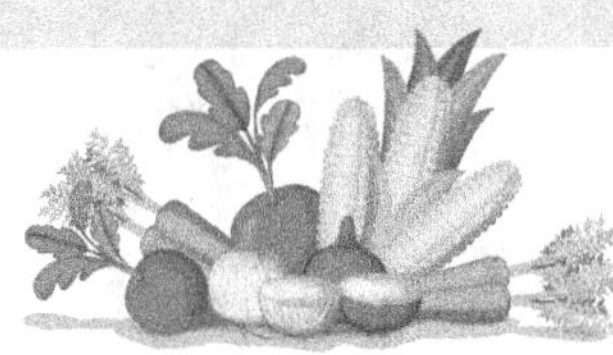 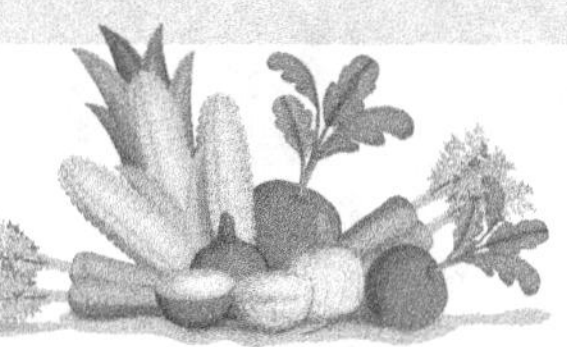

Vegetables
(Choose 3 or More)

Cucumber

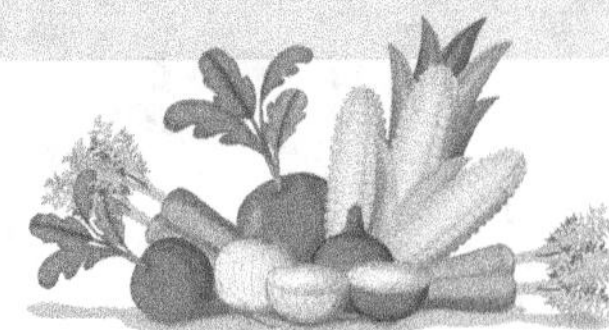 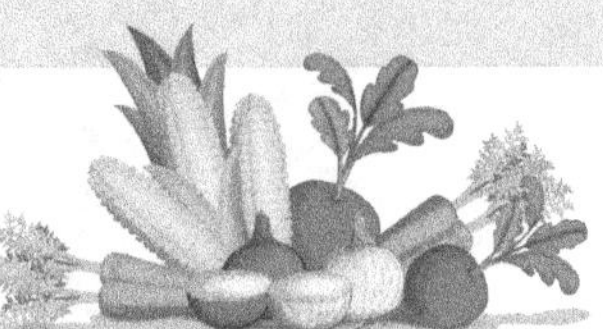

**Vegetables
(Choose 3 or More)**

Kale

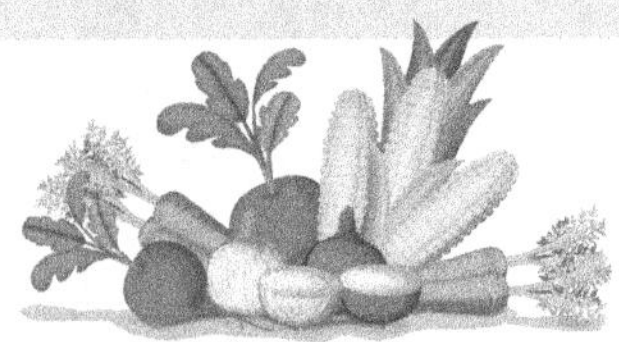 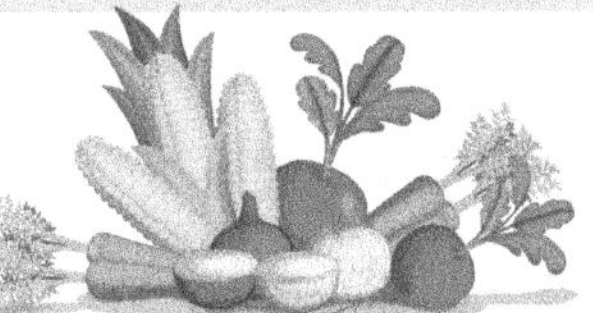

**Vegetables
(Choose 3 or More)**

Beans
(Any Variety)

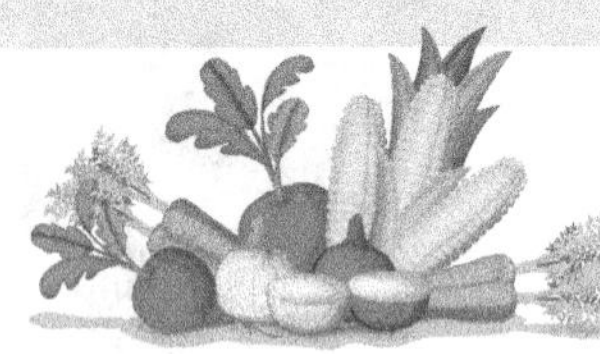 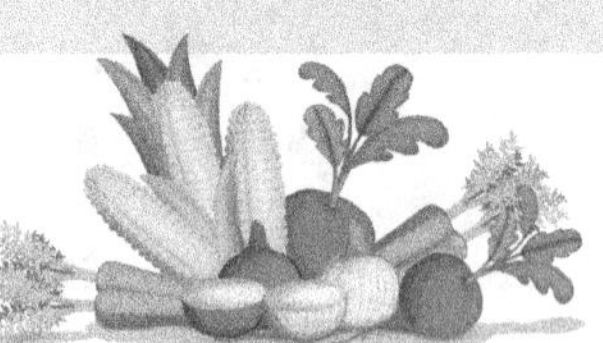

**Vegetables
(Choose 3 or More)**

Spinach

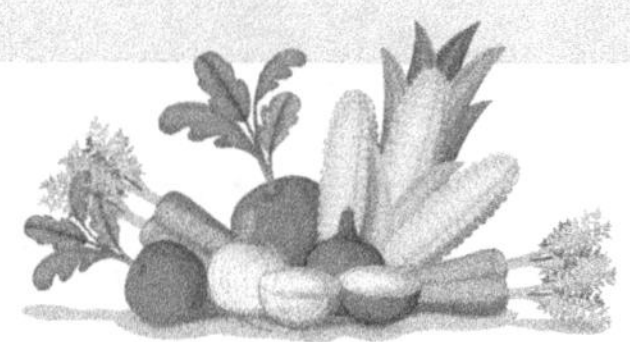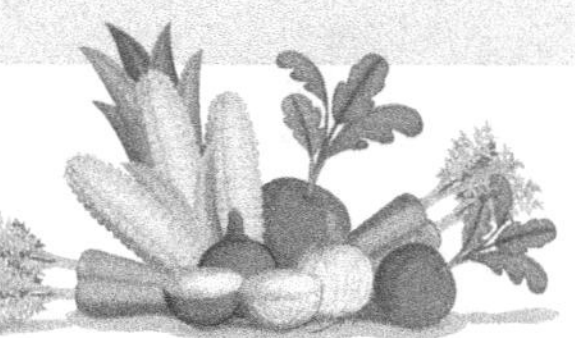

Vegetables
(Choose 3 or More)

Asparagus

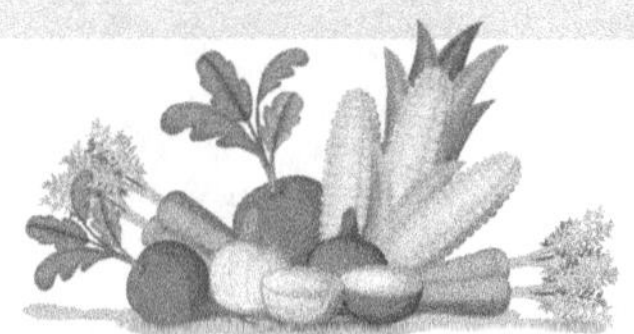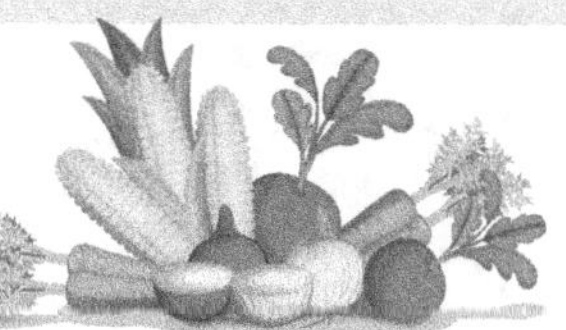

Vegetables
(Choose 3 or More)

Cherry Tomatoes

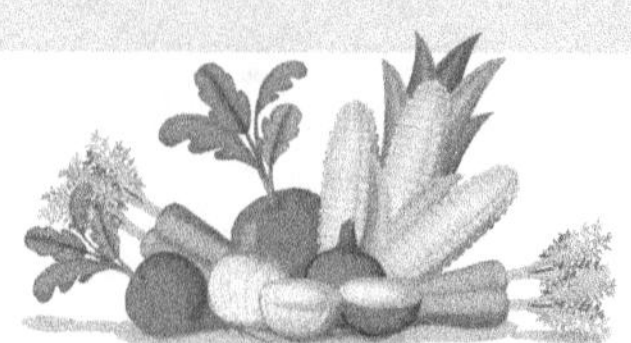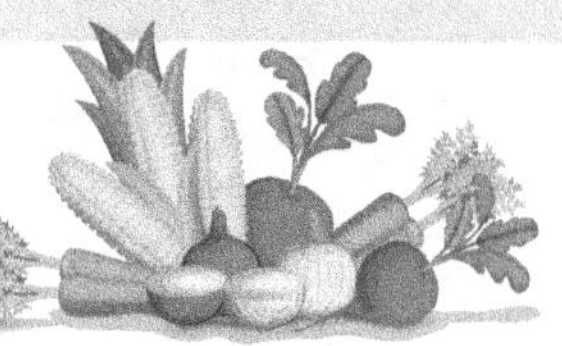

Vegetables
(Choose 3 or More)

Peppers (Any Variety)

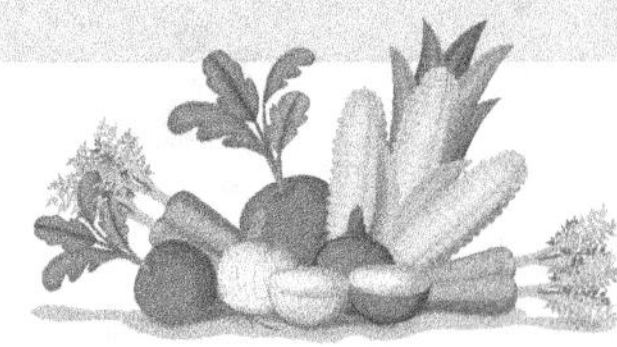 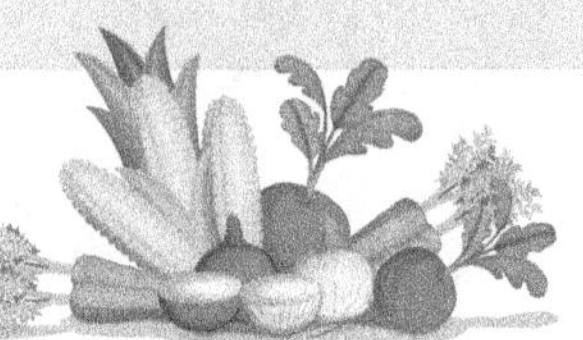

**Vegetables
(Choose 3 or More)**

Avocados

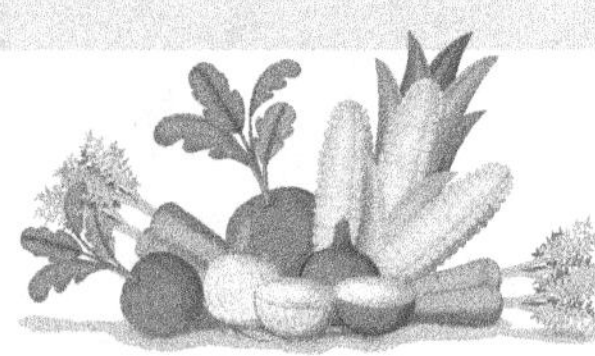 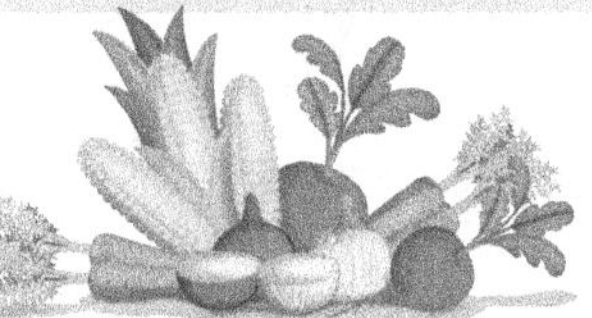

**Vegetables
(Choose 3 or More)**

Sweet Potatoes

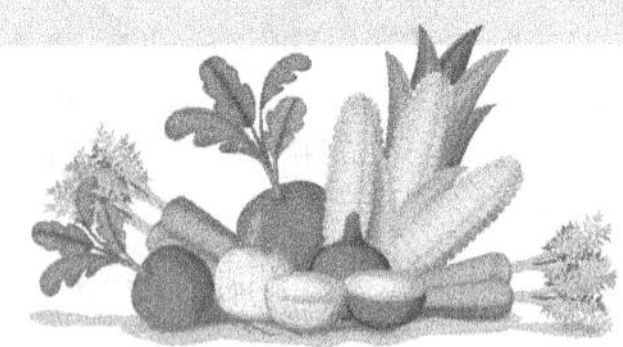 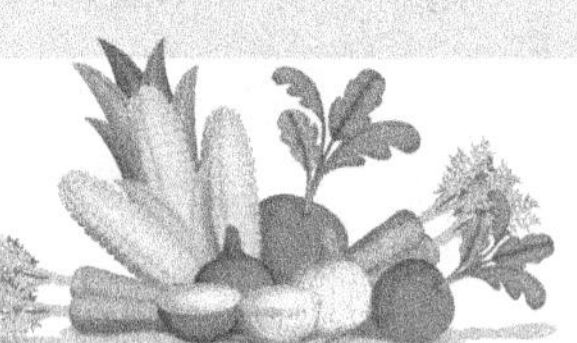

**Vegetables
(Choose 3 or More)**

Green Beans

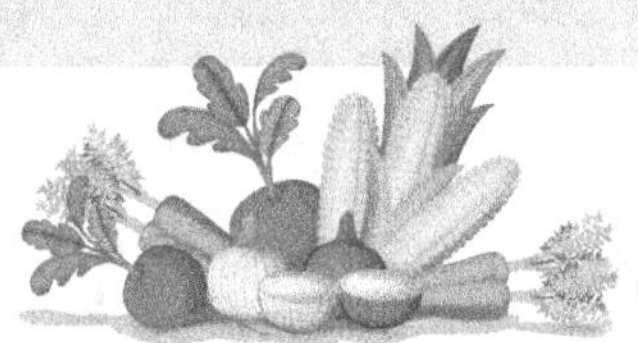 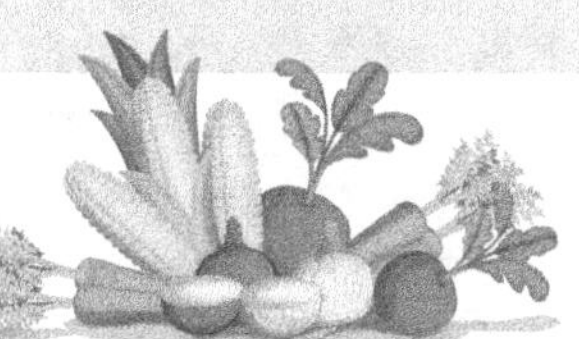

Vegetables
(Choose 3 or More)

Peas

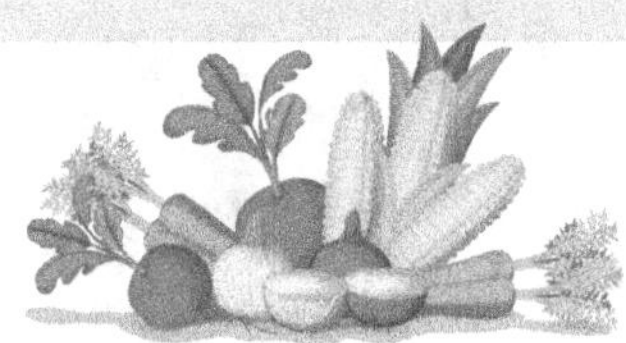 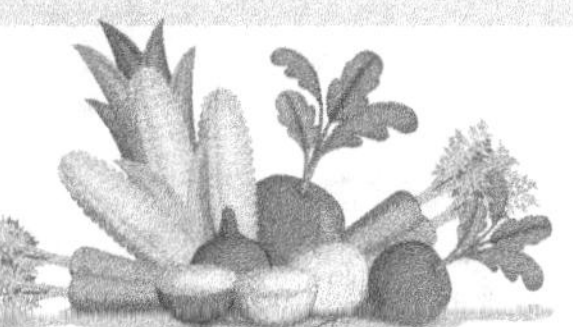

Vegetables
(Choose 3 or More)

Sundried Tomatoes

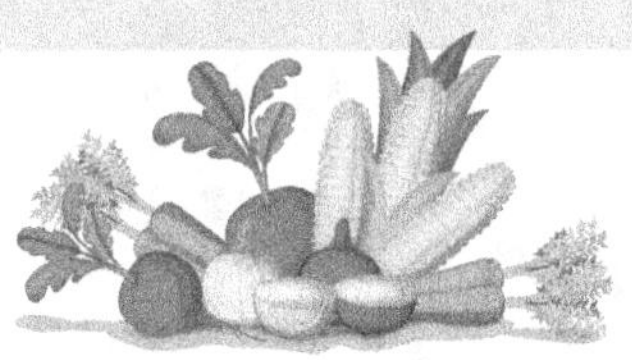 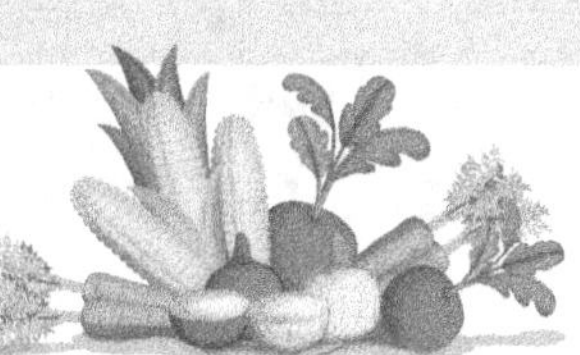

Vegetables
(Choose 3 or More)

Jar of Capers

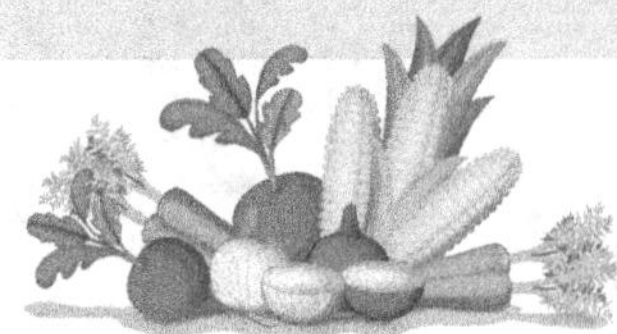 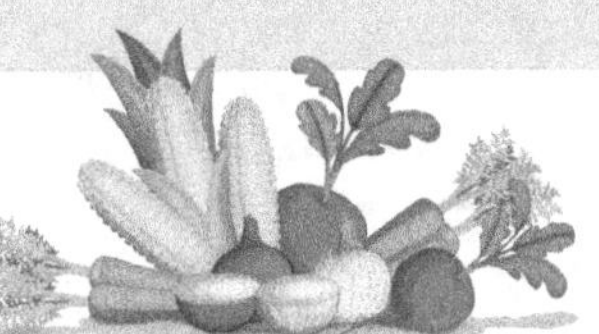

**Vegetables
(Choose 3 or More)**

Carrots

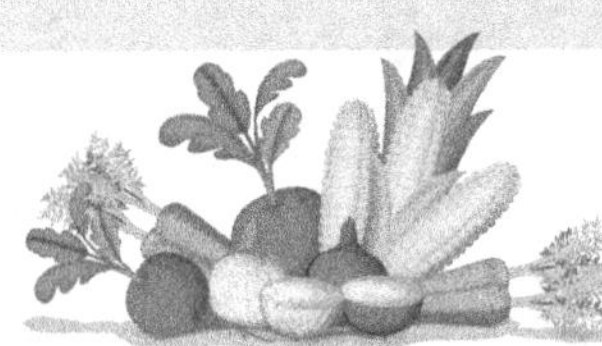 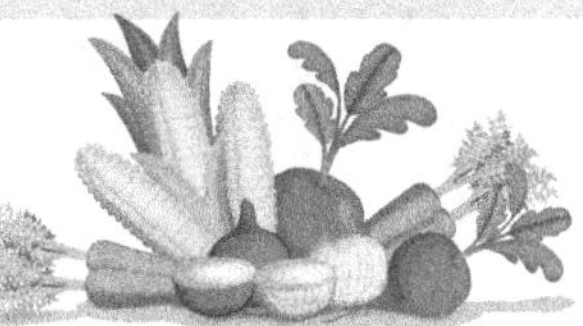

**Vegetables
(Choose 3 or More)**

Roasted Red Peppers

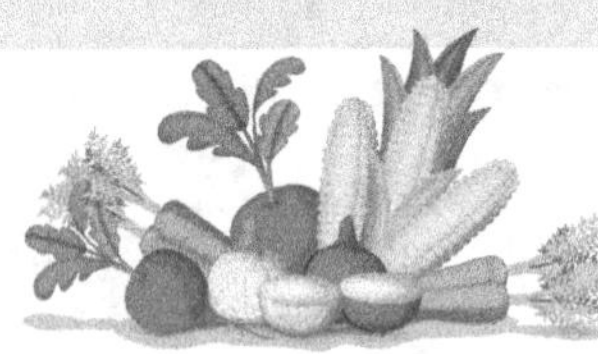 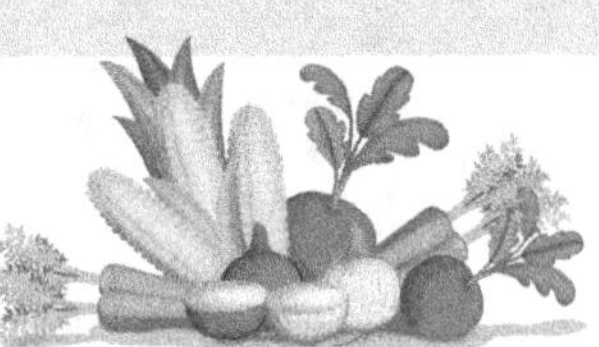

**Vegetables
(Choose 3 or More)**

Squash
(Any Variety)

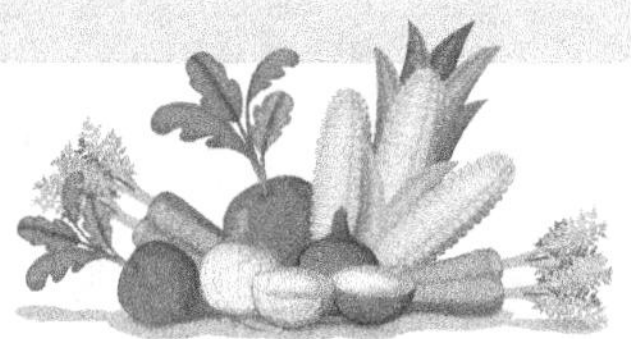 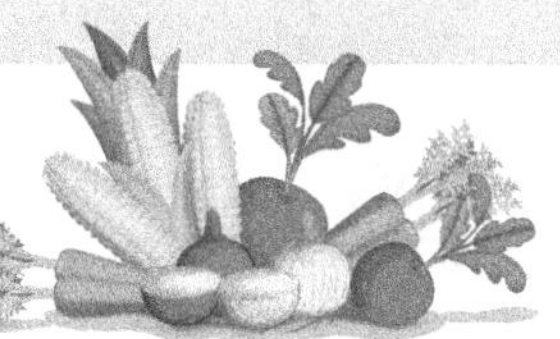

**Vegetables
(Choose 3 or More)**

Cabbage

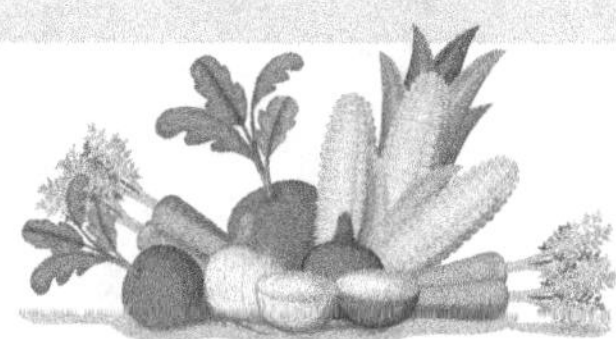 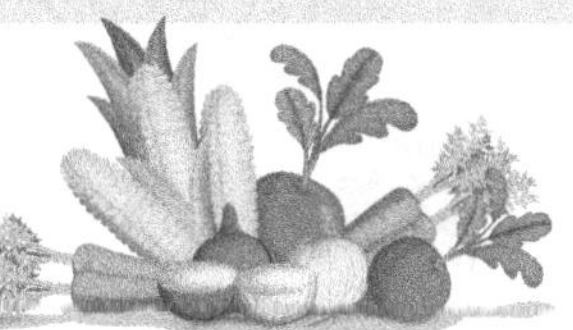

**Vegetables
(Choose 3 or More)**

Slaw Packs (Broccoli, Cabbage, Kale, etc.)

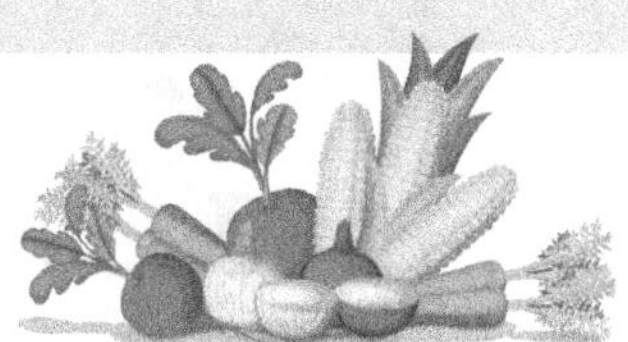 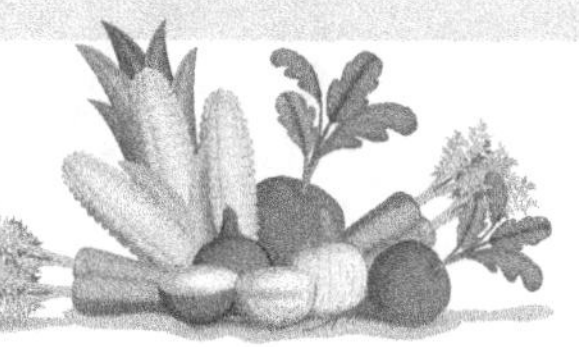

**Vegetables
(Choose 3 or More)**

Cauliflower

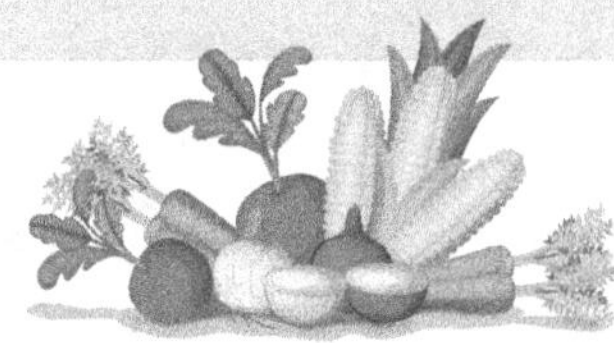 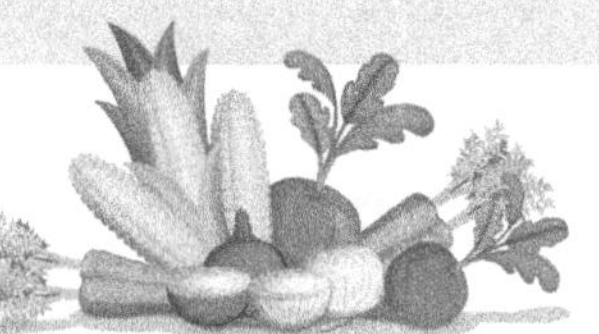

**Vegetables
(Choose 3 or More)**

Brussels sprouts

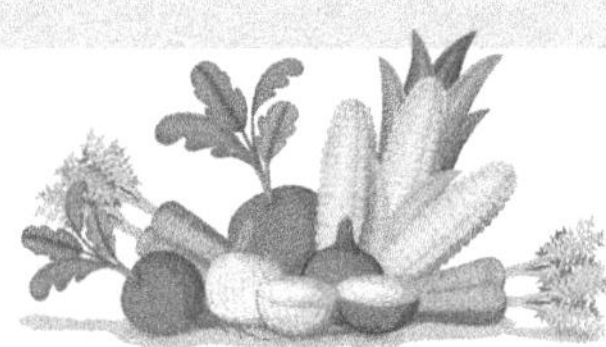 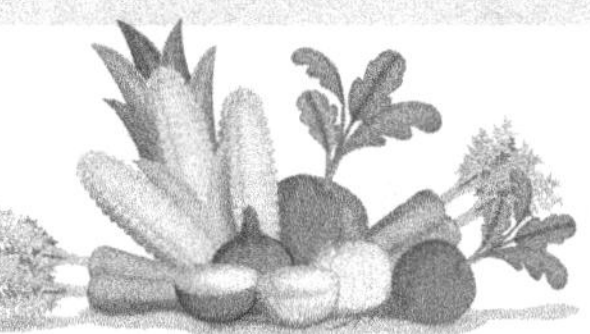

**Vegetables
(Choose 3 or More)**

Frozen Vegetable Mixes

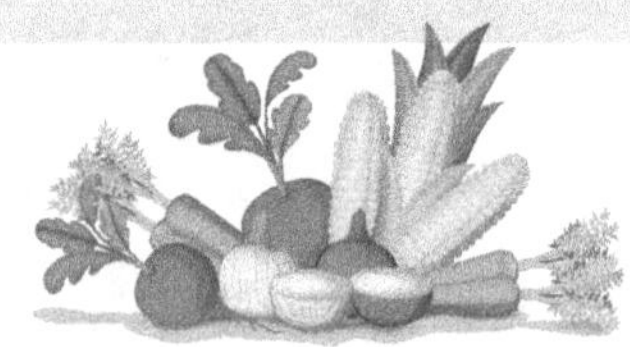 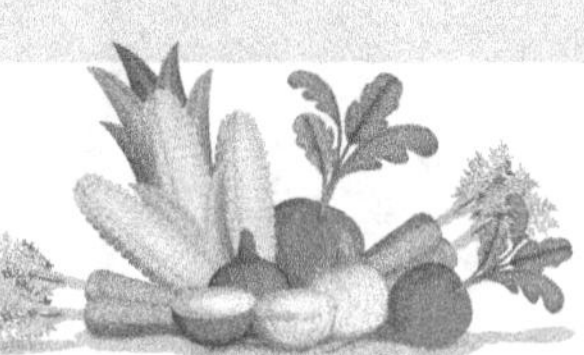

**Vegetables
(Choose 3 or More)**

Mushrooms

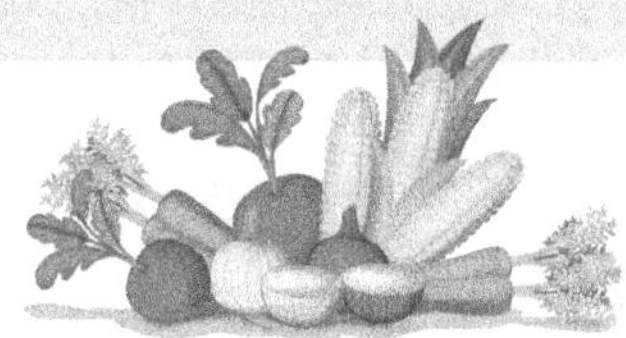 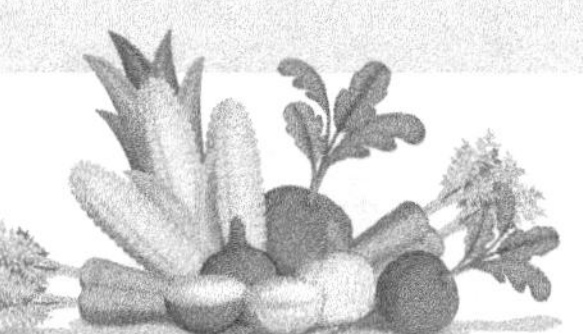

Vegetables
(Choose 3 or More)

Artichokes

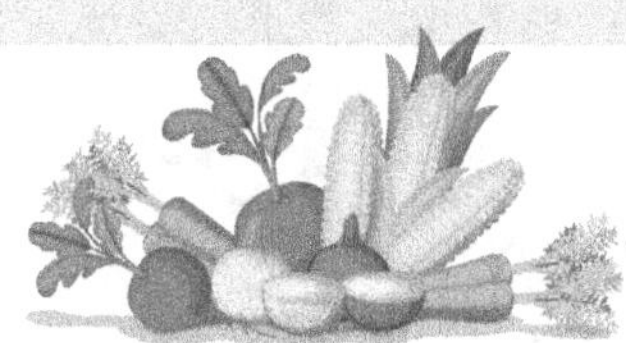 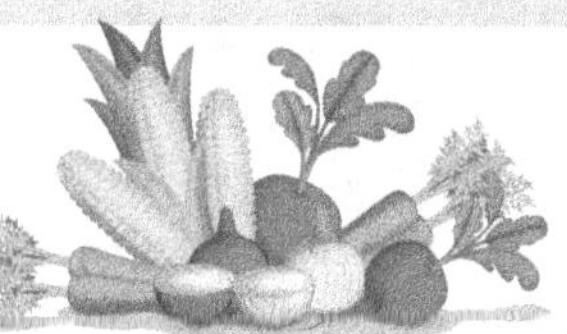

Vegetables
(Choose 3 or More)

Fermented Pickles

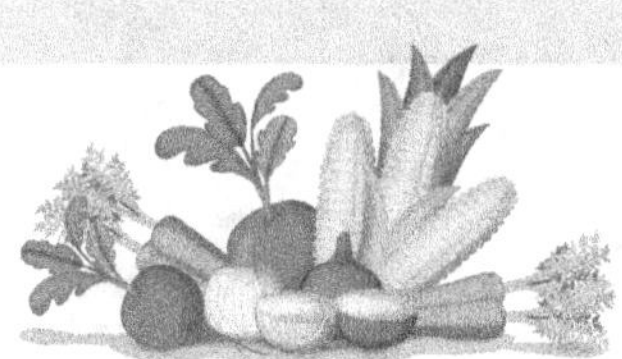 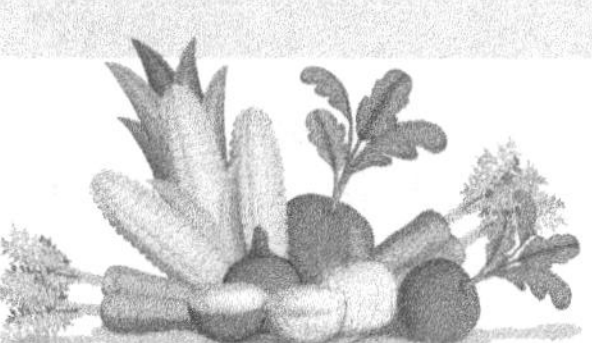

Vegetables
(Choose 3 or More)

Salsa

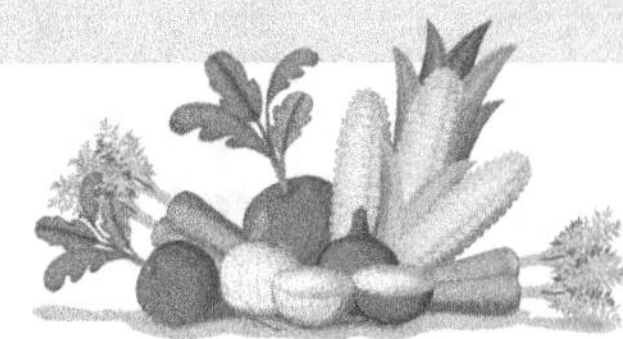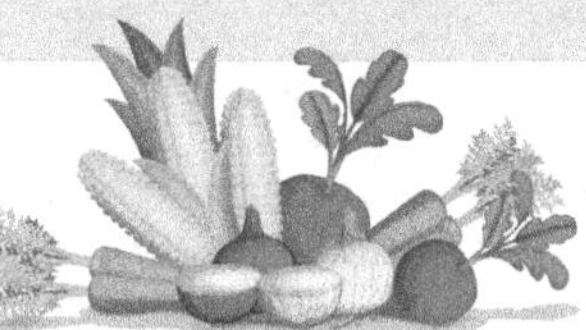

Vegetables
(Choose 3 or More)

Pico Del Gallo

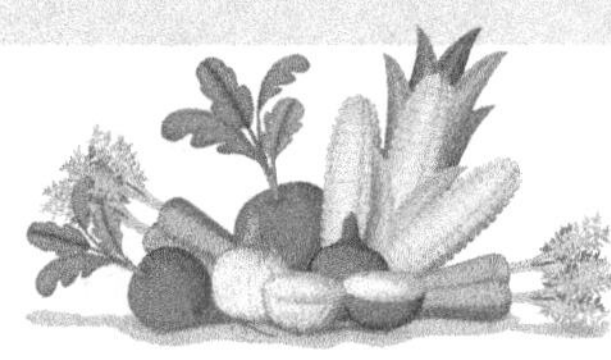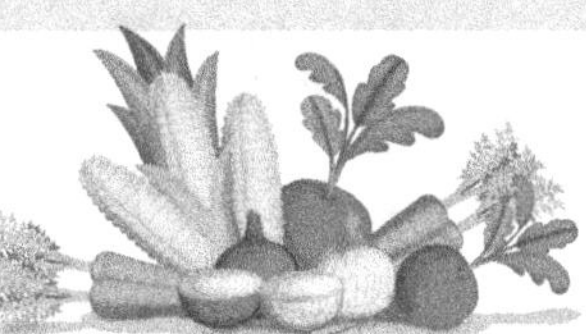

Vegetables
(Choose 3 or More)

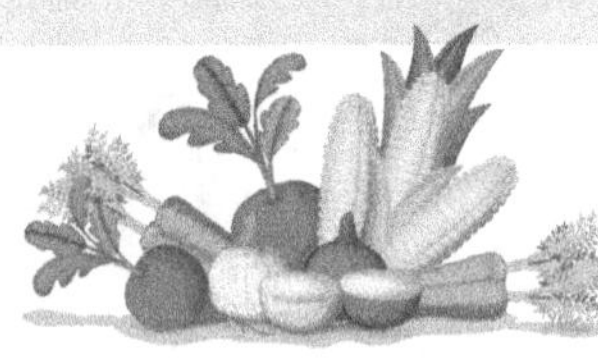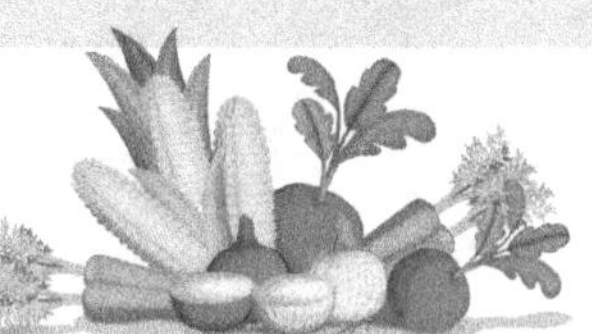

Vegetables
(Choose 3 or More)

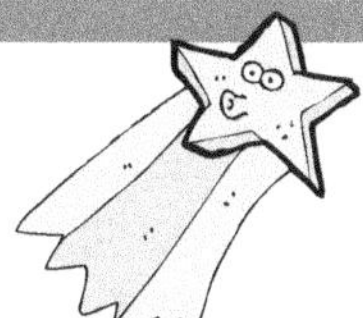 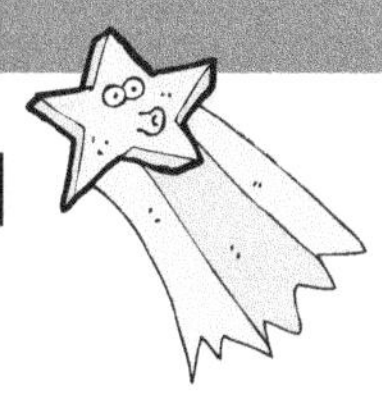

Optional Superfood Add-Ins

Flaxseed

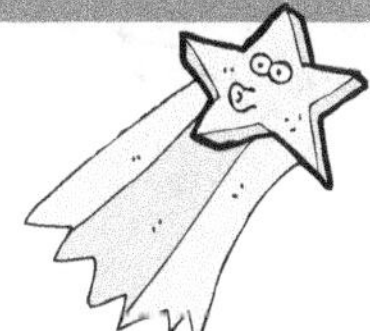 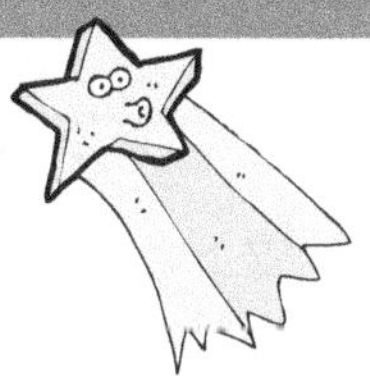

Optional Superfood Add-Ins

Chia Seed

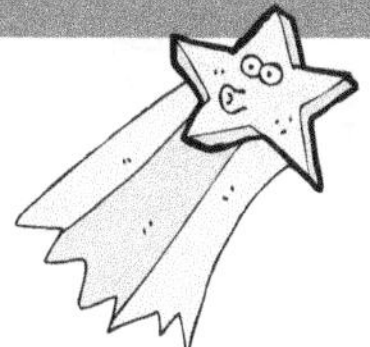 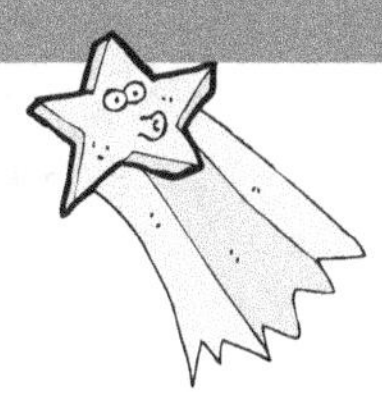

Optional Superfood Add-Ins

Hemp Seed

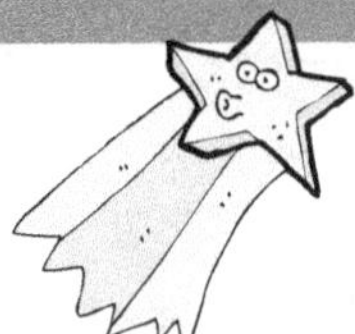 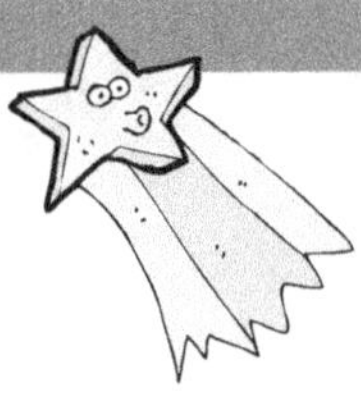

Optional Superfood Add-Ins

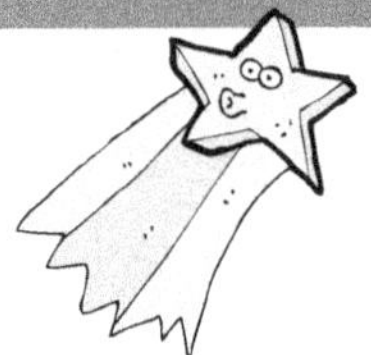 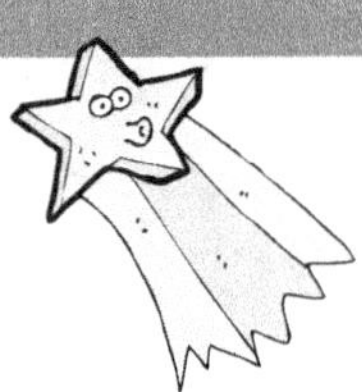

Optional Superfood Add-Ins

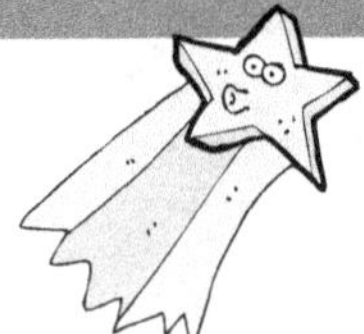 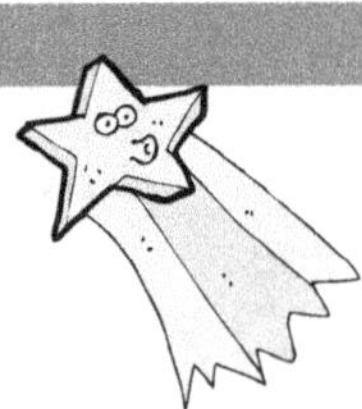

Optional Superfood Add-Ins

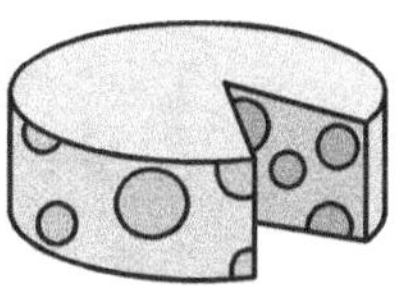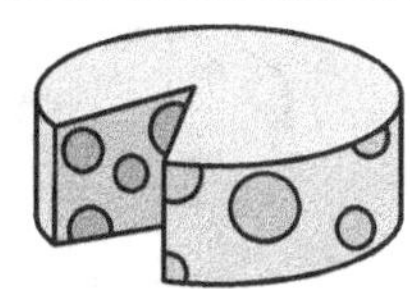

Cheeses (Optional)

Parmesean

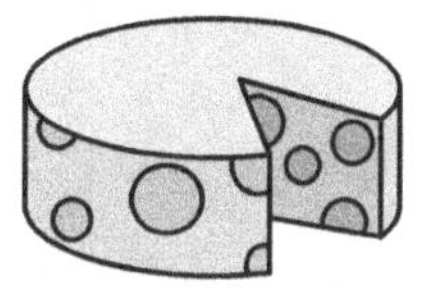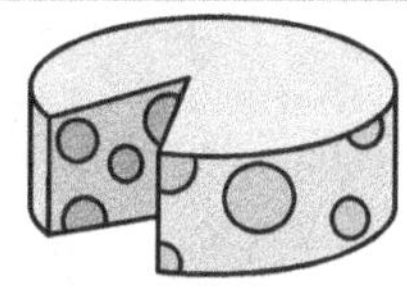

Cheeses (Optional)

Mozzarella

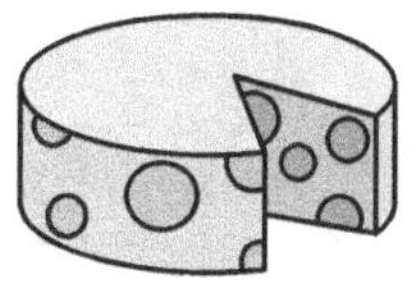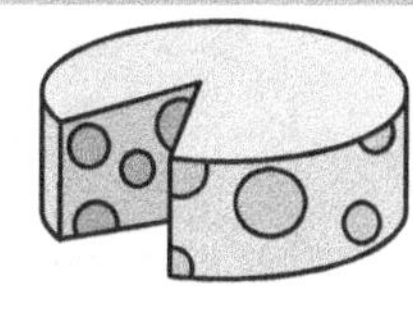

Cheeses (Optional)

Ricotta

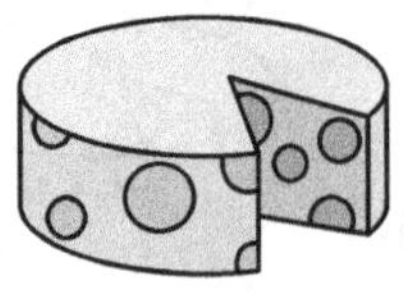 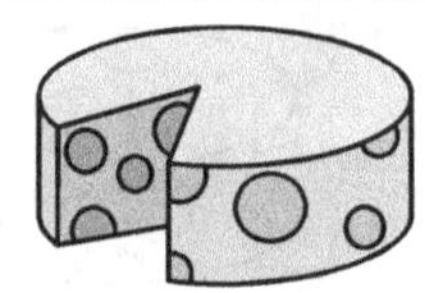

**Cheeses
(Optional)**

Goat

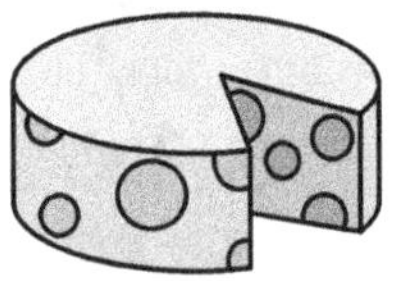 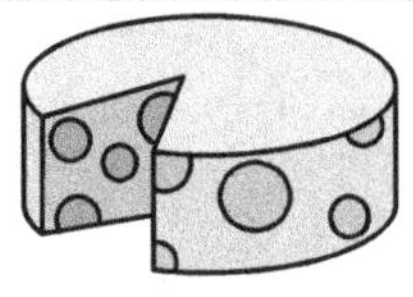

**Cheeses
(Optional)**

Cheddar

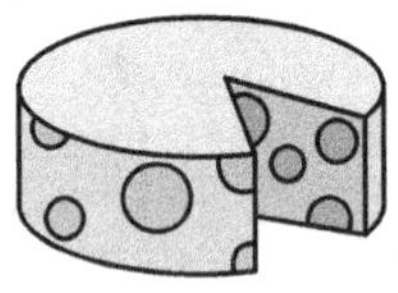 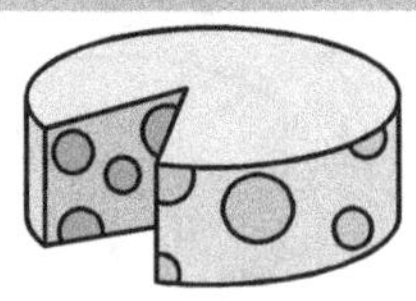

**Cheeses
(Optional)**

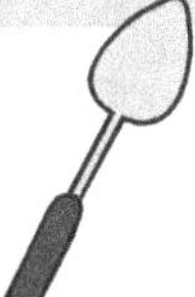

Asian Inspired Seasoning & Sauces
Teriyaki Sauce (Primal Kitchen) or Soy Sauce + choices below:

- Garlic
- Sesame Oil
- Salt
- Black Pepper
- Honey + Ketchup (Primal Kitchen)
- Horseradish
- Rice Vinegar
- Siracha Sauce
- Mirin
- For creamy sauce: Cream Cheese, yogurt; or a can of cream soup
- Asian Vinaigrette
- Chicken/Vegetable Brot

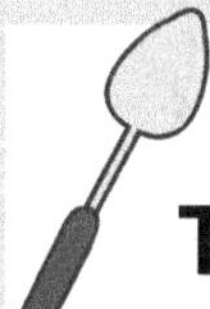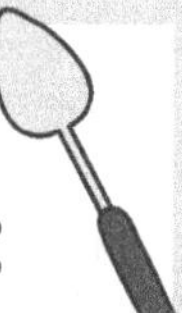

Curry Seasoning & Sauces
Tomato sauce + Honey + Seasonings below:

- Coriander
- Cumin
- Turmeric and Black Pepper
- Garlic
- For creamy sauce: Cream Cheese, yogurt (add after cooking); or a can of cream soup
- Ginger
- Cayenne Pepper
- Mustard
- Curry

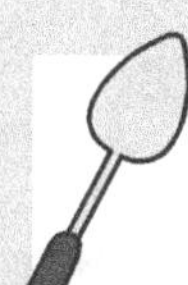

Dressing/Vinagarette Seasoning & Sauces
(Choose 2 or more from 1 card)

- Honey
- Balsamic/Cider Vinegar or Lemon Juice
- Black Pepper
- Chicken Broth/Vegetable broth
- Onion Powder Mix
- Extra Virgin Olive Oil
- Red Pepper Flakes
- Paprika
- White Pepper
- Italian Dressing (I like Primal Kitchen)
- For creamy sauce: Cream Cheese, or yogurt (add after cooking)
- Garlic
- Horseradish

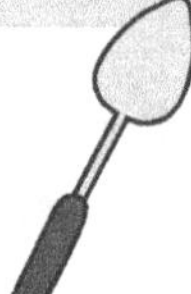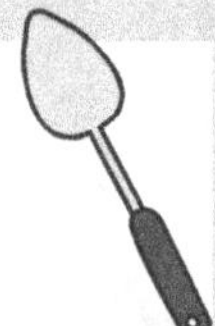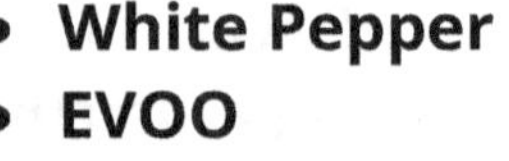

Italian Seasoning & Sauces
(Choose 2 or more from 1 card)

- Montreal Seasoning
- Tomato Sauce
- Italian Seasoning
- Parsley
- Oregano
- Garlic
- Black Pepper
- Salt
- Honey
- Basil
- Sage
- Tomato Soup Can
- For creamy sauce: Cream Cheese, yogurt (add after cooking); or a can of cream soup
- White Pepper
- EVOO

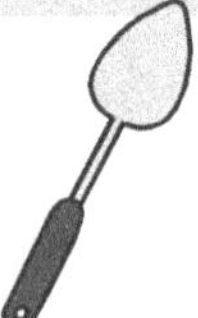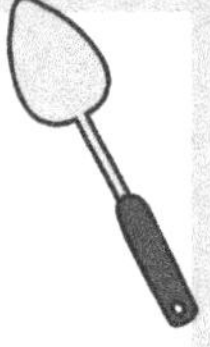

BBQ Seasoning & Sauces
(Choose 2 or more from 1 card)

- Montreal Seasoning
- BBQ Sauce (I like Primal Kitchen)
- White Pepper, Black Pepper, or Cayenne Pepper
- Turmeric and Black Pepper
- Garlic
- Worcestershire Sauce

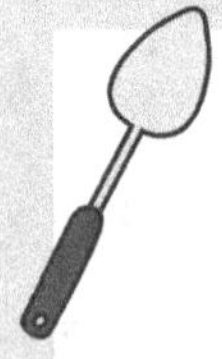

Chili Seasoning & Sauces
(Choose 2 or more from 1 card)

- Black Pepper
- Garlic
- White Pepper
- For creamy sauce: Cream Cheese, yogurt (add after cooking); or a can of cream soup
- Worcestershire Sauce
- Cayenne Pepper
- Montreal Seasoning
- Chili Seasoning
- Chicken/Vegetable broth
- Tomato Sauce
- Salt

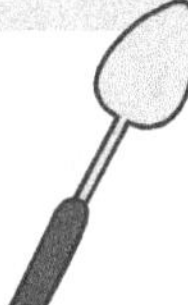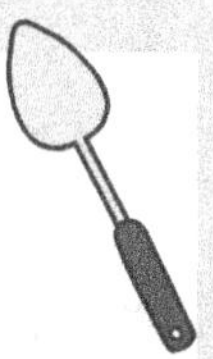

Marinate Inspired Seasoning & Sauces
(Choose 2 or more from 1 card)

- Italian Dressing/Vinaigrette
- White wine sauce
- Garlic
- Caper's
- Lemon juice
- Parsley
- Chicken Broth
- Vegetable Broth
- Black Pepper
- Salt
- Balsamic/Cider Vinegar
- Extra Virgin Olive Oil

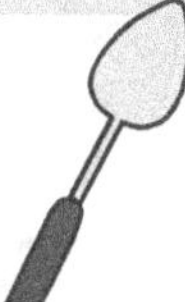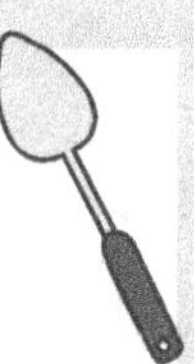

Kickin' "Sausage" Seasoning & Sauces
(Choose 2 or more from 1 card)

- Fennel Seeds
- Garlic
- Paprika
- Black Pepper
- Salt
- White Pepper
- BBQ Sauce
- Worcestershire
- For creamy sauce: Cream Cheese, yogurt (add after cooking); or a can of cream soup

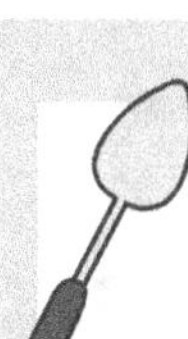

Southwest Inspired Seasoning & Sauces
(Choose 2 or more from 1 card)

- Chipotle Adobe Sauce
- Chicken/ Vegetable Broth
- Taco Seasoning
- Garlic
- Paprika
- Salt
- Lime Juice
- White Pepper
- Lemon Juice
- For creamy sauce: Cream Cheese, yogurt; or a can of cream soup
- Tomato Sauce
- Extra Virgin Olive Oil
- Avocado Oil
- Cilantro

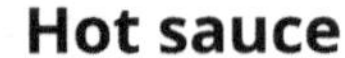

Get Creative Seasoning & Sauces
(Choose 2 or more from 1 card)

- Hot sauce
- Montreal Seasoning
- White wine
- garlic
- Salt
- Black pepper
- White Pepper
- BBQ Sauce
- Onion soup mix
- Turmeric with Black Pepper
- Salad Dressing (I like Primal Kitchen)
- Paprika
- Ranch Packets
- Everything but the Bagel
- Extra Virgin Olive Oil
- Chicken/Veggie broth
- Worcestershire
- For creamy sauce: Cream Cheese, yogurt (add after cooking); or a can of cream soup

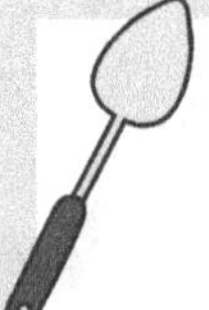

Pesto Seasoning & Sauce
(Choose all on the list, mix in a food processor, Sauté' with ingredients from other cards)

- Basil
- Leafy Green
- Pine Nuts or other nuts
- Parmesan Cheese
- Garlic
- Olive Oil
- Black Pepper
- Salt

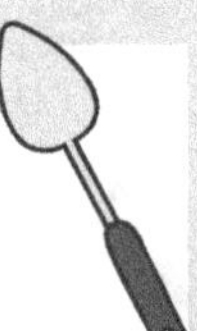

Alfredo Seasoning & Sauce
(Use the Ingredients Below to Make a Healthy Alfredo or simple use Primal Kitchen's Alfredo Sauce)

- Parmesan
- Garlic
- Salt
- Black Pepper

Cream Cheese
Vegetable Broth
Milk (I like 1 % Omega-3 Milk

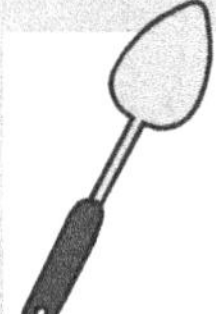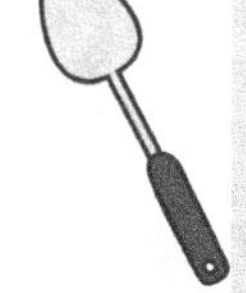

Signature Seasoning & Sauces
(Mix all ingredients below)

- Horseradish
- Avocado or Olive Oil Mayo (I like Primal Kitchen)
- Lemon Juice
- BBQ Sauce (Primal Kitchen)

- Honey
- Siracha Sauce

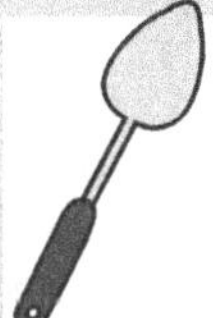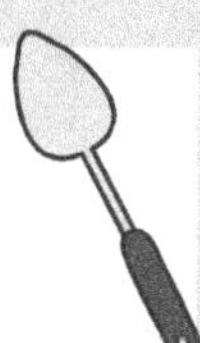

Keep It Simple Seasoning & Sauce

- Pick a Primal Kitchen Sauce or Dressing!

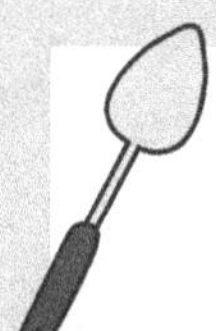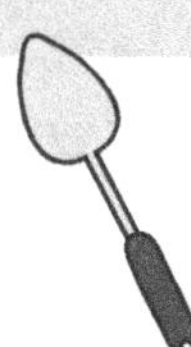

Seasoning & Sauce Combinations

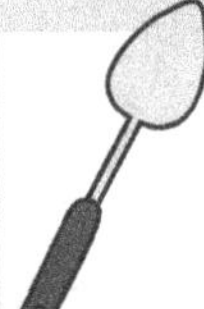 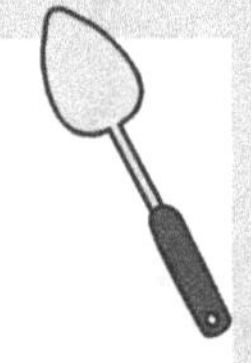

Signature Seasoning & Sauces
(Mix all ingredients below)

- Horseradish
- Avocado or Olive Oil Mayo (I like Primal Kitchen)
- Lemon Juice
- BBQ Sauce (Primal Kitchen)
- Honey
- Siracha Sauce

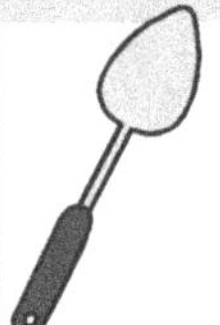 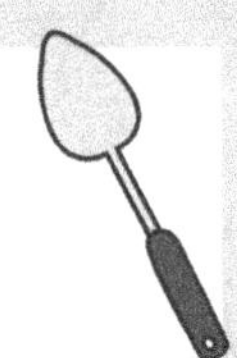

Keep It Simple Seasoning & Sauce

- Pick a Primal Kitchen Sauce or Dressing!

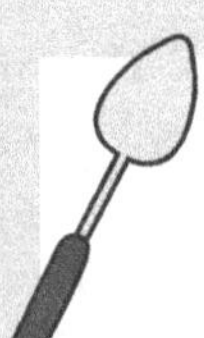 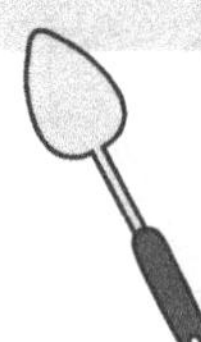

Seasoning & Sauce Combinations

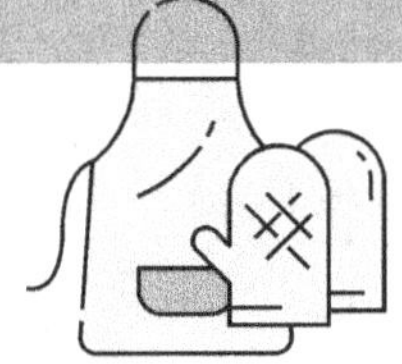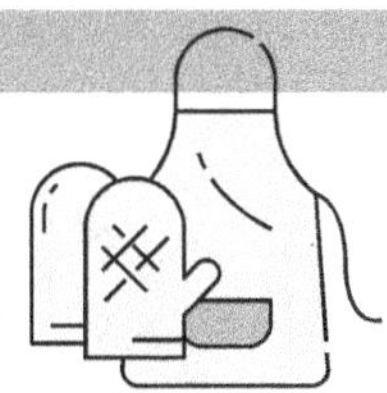

Cooking Methods
(Choose 1 or more)

Sandwich, wrap, lettuce wrap

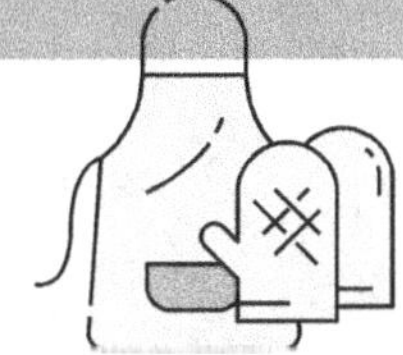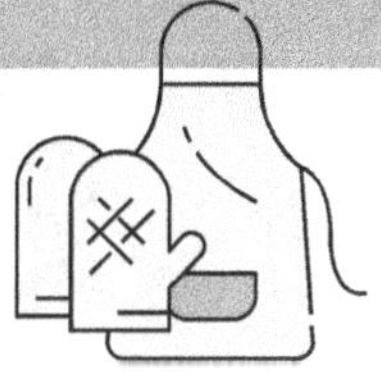

Cooking Methods
(Choose 1 or more)

Dip with chips/crackers

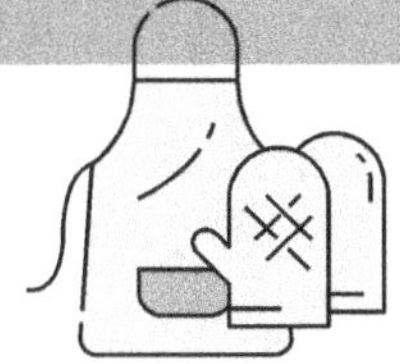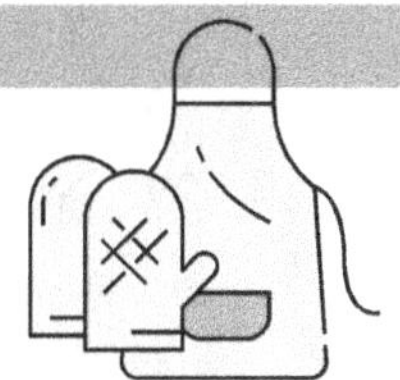

Cooking Methods
(Choose 1 or more)

Salad

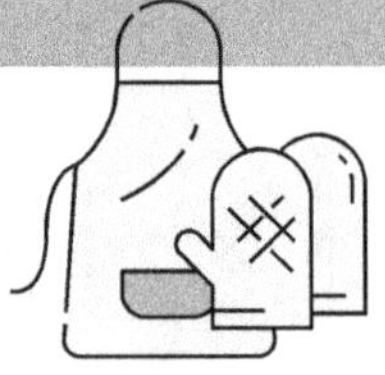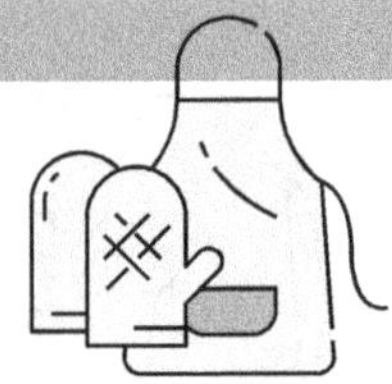

Cooking Methods
(Choose 1 or more)

"Meat"ball/Patty

*Just add egg or flaxseed and water to chosen ingredients and form a ball or patty; bake or sauté

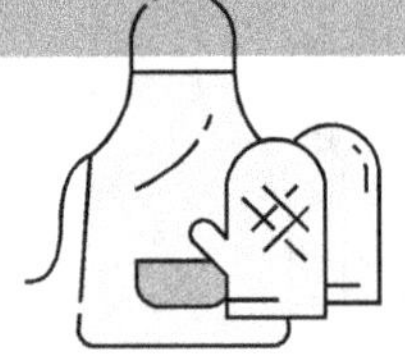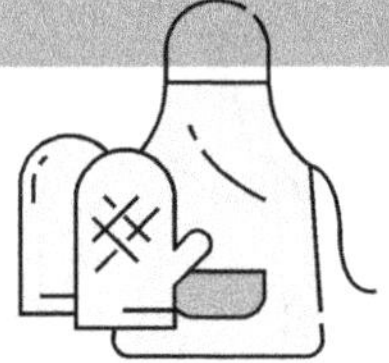

Cooking Methods
(Choose 1 or more)

Saute'

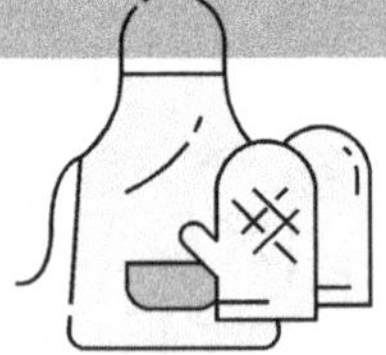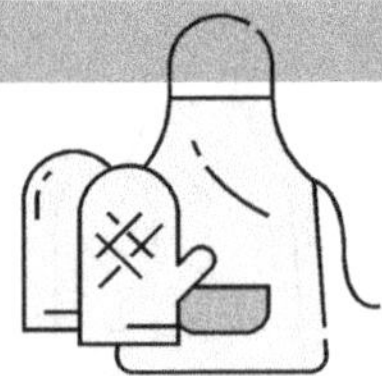

Cooking Methods
(Choose 1 or more)

Bake

Perfect for Mixed and Layered Casseroles

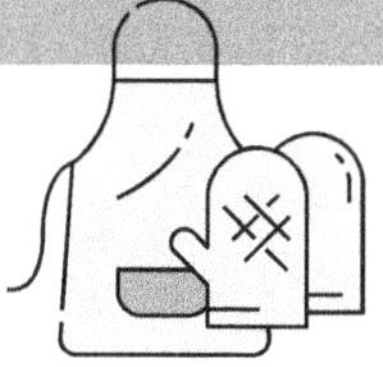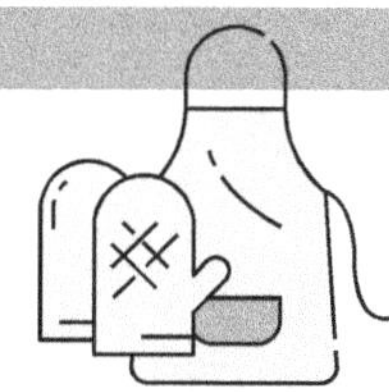

Cooking Methods
(Choose 1 or more)

Slow Cooker

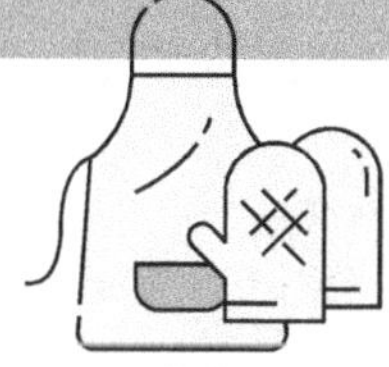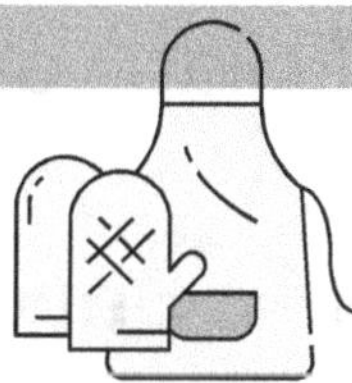

Cooking Methods
(Choose 1 or more)

Pressure Cooker

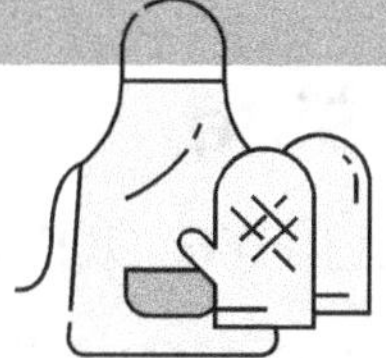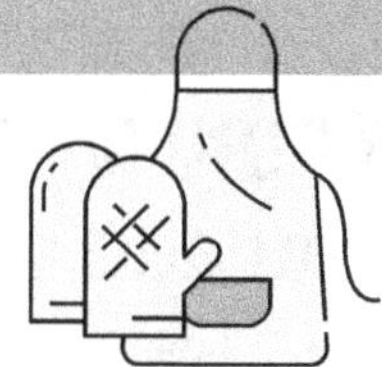

Cooking Methods
(Choose 1 or more)

Egg Muffin Cups

Add eggs and ingredients of your choice to a muffin cup and bake.

Chapter 7:
Snacks and Sides

You are almost there! You can now make super easy meals without the mental stress of planning. The final step is figuring out what kinds of sides and snacks you would like to keep in your house.

With snacks and sides, you have an easy opportunity to get in some of those foods (like from fruits and berries) that don't always fit into your meals as well.

Fruits as a Snack or Side
Fruits and vegetables are about the healthiest snack or side you can get! In fact, they are probably one of the best choices when it comes to snacks! Remember, fruits are packed with antioxidants, vitamins, minerals, and filling fiber. Plus, fruits are low in calories so eating fruits can aid in weight loss. Fruits like bananas, apples, oranges, grapes, and fruit cups or pre-portioned mixed fruit containers make perfect on-the-go snacks.

Fruit, Yogurt, and Granola as a Snack or Side
When you add yogurt to your fresh fruits, you are getting all of the above benefits of fruit PLUS probiotics and protein!

And Remember, according to research probiotics may:
Support Digestive heath
Support immune function
Have anti-inflammatory properties
Help with mood and mood disorders like depression, anxiety, stress
Reduce cognitive decline and the risk of Alzheimer's and Dementia
May aid in addiction recovery
Promote a healthy heart

Vegetables as your Snack or Side
Remember diets high in fruits and vegetables have been shown to reduce the risk of all sorts of diseases and conditions like Alzheimer's, Dementia, heart disease, stroke, and cancer. In fact, the diets of people who live in the Blue Zones mostly consist of beans, legumes, fruits, vegetables, nuts, and whole grains. So if we want to have a diet that more closely resembles the Blue Zones, we should be incorporating more vegetables (and fruits, whole grains, nuts, and legumes) into our meals AND snacks! Raw vegetables make a great on-the-go gluten free and nut free snack. You can pair them with hummus to get some added protein!

Whole fruits and vegetables are fantastic options for sides and snacks, but sometimes you may need or want a packaged snack option. Deciding which packaged snacks are nutrient dense and less processed can be overwhelming, and remember we are trying to reduce our mental load!

If making snack selections is frustrating for you, or if you wish you had a list of healthy packaged snack ideas in one place, please take the time to check out my healthy packaged snacks collections *on our blog.*

On these lists I have included protein, probiotic, omega-3, antioxidant, vitamin, mineral, whole grain, and fiber-rich packaged snacks as well as nut free and gluten free options.

Chapter 8:
A Healthy, Happy, Meaningful Life with the Help of Mindfulness

I hope and pray that I was able to adequately explain in this book, how nutrition can help you live a healthier, happier, more meaningful life. We want to be as healthy as we can so that we have the energy to serve God and others, have a mind ready to learn what God want us to discover, and have as positive a mood as possible. After all, we tend to show kindness more when we are in a good mood.

But Mindfulness can help with our moods, behaviors, and even our health as well! The benefits of mindfulness can not be overstated.

In fact, mindfulness techniques are so beneficial that schools have even started implementing mindfulness programs. Although more research is needed, current research indicates that implementing Mindfulness programs in schools may improve social behaviors, mood, stress levels, and even academic performance and test scores. Schools are even reporting less suspensions, detentions, violent incidences, principal visits, bullying, and classroom disruptions since incorporating mindfulness programs!

Benefits of Mindfulness

If you think about it, these results make since, don't they? Practicing mindfulness techniques can relieve stress and help us have better self-control. When we have less stress and learn to have more self-control, we tend to make better choices. Less ideal choices can sometimes cause even more stress, which brings us full circle. Furthermore, aren't we better able to focus and learn when our brains are calm verses stressed? Mindfulness can help with stress and promote a more positive outlook on life. Less stress and more positivity promote better health. It's all beautifully related.

So you can see how mindfulness activities can be so impactful, but for me, the most profound impact happens when I combine faith and mindfulness.

One aspect of mindfulness is about focusing on being present. But with faith-based mindfulness, you are focusing on how God is present with you in that very moment, and while focusing on God's presence you get to notice all the gifts from God and the beautiful little things in God's world.

Remember when I mentioned that my goals are to serve God and others and love the people around me as best I can?

Well I actually have a little more detailed Goal List:

1.   My greatest desire is to glorify God in all that I do. I want to show God's love through kindness and giving. My prayer is that I listen for God's guidance in every situation because when I listen to God, amazing things happen, and I WANT TO BE AMAZED!!!

2. I wish to have a peaceful and positive life and a grateful attitude. I want to enjoy the little moments by taking the time to notice God's world and soak it up!

3. We humans seem to have a natural desire to work and create. We want to have meaning and purpose in our lives. This is true for me too. In my ideal life, I want to learn, grow, and work. I want to create something new, and in some small way make the world better. I want to challenge my mind through reading and learning from God and others, and I want to challenge my body through physical activity.

4. Just as I desire to work, grow, and be challenged, I equally want to have time to rest, relax, and play. Sometimes finding the time to relax is the most difficult challenge in life, and yet so important for our health and our ability to serve God and others.

5. I want to serve God and others and love the people around me the best I can.

Faith-based mindfulness helps me fulfill that list like nothing else.

Here is how my life has been transformed through faith-based mindfulness:

- I listen to God more. Listening to God helps me make better choices. I'm not letting negative emotions take control of my actions. (At least not as often, anyway)
- Now I am more at peace and comforted because I am noticing God is with me everywhere.
- I get to have more goose-bump-"I'm awe struck" moments because when I intentionally focus on God in the present moment, I actually see what God is doing in my life and the lives of others around me. By focusing on God in the present moment, I get to experience the feeling of amazement more often, and, again, I WANT TO BE AMAZED!!! (Don't we all want to be beautifully amazed?)

Mindful Eating: The Prayer Before a Meal That Stops Me from Over Eating and Other Mindful Eating Techniques

Did you know learning to pause and pray is what finally helped me (a dietitian) stop overeating! This pausing and praying is one of the mindful eating techniques discussed in this chapter. When you mindfully eat, you get to experience ALL these faith-based mindfulness benefits and more.

Mindful eating gives us the opportunity to focus on God's presence, feel gratitude for God's gift of food, and rest our brain! We get to have mini mindfulness moments with God EVERY. TIME. WE. EAT!

With mindful breathing, we are pausing and centering out minds on one thing- breathing. When we are mindfully eating, we are still pausing and centering our brain on one thing, but this time that one thing is eating. With faith-based mindful eating, we are resting our brain by focusing on God and the food God provided.

Some of the other benefits to mindful eating are:

WEIGHT LOSS

I don't want to focus too much on this because all sizes can be healthy. Some people are naturally smaller and some naturally weigh more. We have different builds and genetics. Plus, other things like medications, medical conditions, and even uncontrollable seasons in life can affect weight.

But I also don't want you to feel that wanting to lose weight is somehow wrong. You may want to see if weight loss will help you have more energy or help with a medical condition. Maybe you feel like you could keep up with your children more if you carried less weight or maybe you want to see if weight loss can help with joint pain.

There are reasons you may desire weight loss, and fortunately mindful eating can help with weight loss while also helping you stop that food obsessing often associated with dieting.   Mindful eating helps you feel full and notice your hunger/satiety cues. Moreover, the desire to binge decreases because you are actually enjoying your food ALL THE TIME.

Although, mindful eating is so much more than weight loss and weight loss is not the general focus, I still want you to know all the possible outcomes of mindful eating and one outcome can be weight loss. In fact, I lost 50 pounds, myself, through mindful eating!

RELIEVES STRESS

Like the mindfulness practices above, Mindful eating is a stress reliever. Making time for mediation or quiet time can help reduce stress, but when you are super busy you can make eating a time to de-stress through mindful eating. Mindfulness is about slowing down and calming your brain. When you meditate you center your thoughts. When you mindfully eat, you center your thoughts on eating. You try to focus on eating and nothing else. You eat slowly and taste your food. In other words, mindful eating is a time to de-stress in a busy world.

Did you know that stress feeds harmful bacteria in our gut? Stress, alone, can cause inflammation, decrease immune function, cause weight gain, and increase your risk for many chronic conditions so you can see, yet again, how mindful eating promotes a healthy mind, body, and spirit.

MAY REDUCE THE RISK OF MANY CHRONIC CONDITIONS

Mindful eating can aid in digestion. How? Although most digestive enzymes are released in the stomach, digestion actually starts in the mouth. One enzyme, called Salivary Amylase, is released in the mouth. This enzyme starts breaking down carbohydrates. In fact, if you let a piece of bread sit in your mouth for a moment, you may notice a sweeter taste. That taste occurs because the more complex carbohydrate is breaking down into a simpler sugar. Chewing thoroughly helps with digestion because digestion starts in the mouth! Plus, chewing thoroughly gives the enzymes in your stomach more surface area to do their work, which again promotes healthy digestion and absorption.

Mindful Eating and Gut Health

These reasons, along with the ability to relieve stress, are how mindful eating can aid in digestion. Remember, poor gut health is related to inflammation and reduced immune function. Gut health, inflammation, and immunity are all linked to many condition including IBS, Crohn's, Autoimmune Disease, Alzheimer's, heart disease, stroke, brain function and focus, mood and even depression and anxiety, to name a few. So anything that promotes a healthy gut is something worth looking into in my book. (Fortunately, a mindful eating guide IS included in my book!)

Do you remember those astonishing people from the Blue Zones? Interestingly, along with following similar diet patterns, the people in these Blue Zone tend to naturally practice mindful eating and are in tune with their hunger as well! Hmm, perhaps they really are onto something!

A Note on Adequate Mindful Sleep and Exercise

Sleep

Turns out adequate sleep and exercise are important for our mental health and brain function as well. Inactivity and inadequate quantity and quality of sleep can increase your risk of many of these chronic conditions as well! Again, it is all connected and each aspect affects the other. For example, practicing mindfulness before bed can help with sleep. Certain foods can also help you feel calm and get better sleep as well, which is another way nutrition can help reduce the risk of medical conditions and improve moods.

Sleep can also help with the following:

- Sleep gives the cleansing wave time to occur. The cleansing wave is a muscular contraction that helps clear debris from the small intestines. The cleansing wave only happens when we are not digesting like when we sleep. (Waiting to eat between meals can help with this as well)
- Improves immune function
- Improves energy levels and fatigue
- Helps with mood and mood disorders such as depression. Anxiety, stress
- Improves brain function, focus, and attention
- Aids in weight management (lack of sleep can cause weight gain)
- Reduces the risk of heart disease and stroke

Exercise

Exercise doesn't have to be running on a treadmill, although it can be. Just being active and moving throughout the day can do wonders for the mind, body, and spirit. Take the Blue Zone residents, for example. They are naturally active throughout the day. They maintain gardens, clean the house, and walk to their destinations. They are rarely sitting. These people also live social lives, and tend to spend time in fellowship with others instead of just being on their phones.

Mindfulness can be incorporated to both sleep and exercise. Mindful breathing can help relax your mind and body and help you get to sleep. And exercise will be more enjoyable when you focus on the present instead of thinking about all that you have to do when you finish your workout.

What Does a Mindful Day Look Like?

Mindfulness is about being in the present moment. The past is gone and the future has not happened, but the present is HERE and NOW.

Think about it. What do we spend most of our time stressing and worrying about?…The past and the future. Think about how much less stress we would have if we learned to focus on the present moment.

Mindful eating is about focusing on eating and enjoying every bite. Mindful living is about focusing and enjoying whatever you are doing in that moment. Mindfulness is also about having a grateful approach to life. When we are mindflully living, we focus on the positive and what we are thankful for in the present moment. For me, mindfulness is about focusing on God's presence in our lives at every moment and focusing on the beauty in God's world. Sounds simple right? Yeah, I know. It is a lot easier said than done. Sometimes we will still worry about the past and future, but fortunately mindfuless techniques can help us live in the present a little more often.

Hopefully we have established the characteristics of mindfulness, but how do we incorporate mindfulness into our daily lives?

A Mindful Day Might Look Like This:

1. Pause, Breath, and Pray Before Entering a New Place

Pause…take a moment to breath and mindfully pray before entering a new environment and before eating. We will talk more about the prayer before eating later, but for now let's focus on the pause before entering a new environment.

When I pray, I ask God to help me remember to show love and kindness in this current environment. I then thank God for being with me, and I pray that I hear and mindfully listen for God's guidance while I am in this place. So pausing and praying before entering a new environment means, I pray on the way to my kids school, before entering the grocery store, or before entering my friend's house, or going to a park. I pray before a family reunion or a meeting at work.

Another great place to pause and pray is at a red light. Instead of feeling impatient and bored while waiting for the light to change, try taking deep breaths and praying. Use the red light as a time to relax and be present. By doing this, we remember God is with us everywhere. By pausing, breathing, and praying, we can better focus on the moment and on God in every place.

This act helps keep us calm and comforted and helps us react in a more loving way in different situations.

This one pause was not only crucial for my nutritional health, but also in every aspect of my life. Yes, I pause before meals, but I also found that pausing before every new situation was crucial to my behavior, actions, and mood.

1 Thessalonians 5:16-18 talks about praying continuously. In a way, this pause thoughout my day and before eating helps me pray more continuously.

But there is more. I also paused when I was feeling a strong emotion. I began to notice the importance of pausing and praying when I felt angry, or before saying something difficult, or before even talking with my children.

I noticed the importance of not only pausing and praying before meals and snacks, but also before bed and before getting up in the morning. When I forget to do this, I noticed the difference in MY actions and my strength to endure life.

On the days that I do a better job of pausing, I notice God's presence and God's guidance more. When I pause more, I feel like I am truly letting God lead me, and I am reminded that no matter what happens,God is right there. I can feel God's presence in the very room with me, and I feel I have the strength to focus on God's will instead of my emotions. We don't have to rush into every situation, and we don't have to rush to speak. We can and should PAUSE and take our time in life.

2. Use Your Senses to Focus on the People and the Place

Once you have entered each new environment, place, or building, the next step is to focus on the people and the place you are in. In other words, use your senses to be present in the moment instead of thinking about all the things you have to do later. This is particularly important to me when I am with my children. Worrying about all that I have to do, doesn't help me, and I miss out on beautiful moments with my kids.Why worry about things you can't do anything about at that moment?

.

This is a hard one, but one we should continue to strive to achieve. I recently caught myself worrying instead of being present with my child. I was late for a meeting, and I was waiting on my daughter's teacher to arrive so that I could leave for the meeting. While I was impatiently waiting, my 4-year-old daughter was twirling and giggling. I suddenly realized that I was missing out on what was right in front of me. I couldn't do anything about being late so why should I worry?

At that moment, I stopped worrying and started twirling and giggling with my daughter. This moment of waiting ended up being a beautiful, special moment, all because I chose to live in the moment.

3. Practice Gratitude (There are Actual Exercises that Can Help!)

When we approach life with a grateful attitude and look for the good in life, the benefits are endless. According to *"Time Special Edition Mindfulness: The New Science of Health and Happiness,"* gratitude practices have been associated with improved kidney function, reduction in blood pressure, decreased stress hormones, increased energy levels, and increased reports of happiness. When we focus on the positive aspects of life, we tend to have more compassion and kindness for others; thus, the circle of positivity continues. Now the person you showed kindness to may leave feeling more grateful and positive. Now they will be more likely to pass it on.

Do you know you can do some things that can help you have a more grateful attitude?

Gratitude Techniques:

Keep a gratitude journal is a helpful gratitude technique. Every night, write down what you were thankful for that day. Again, according to *"Time Special Edition Mindfulness: The New Science of Health and Happiness,"* even this small exercise is also helpful.

Don't want to even write? Try this… You remember that moment you pause and pray before entering a new place? While you are praying, remember to thank God for something as well.

4.Making Time for Quiet Time

We all need to rest. We need time to clear our thoughts and feel the weight of responsibility lifted for a little while. When I take time to just relax in God's presence, it feels like a chance to completely be myself with the only One who loves me unconditionally. The problems of the world are gone for a moment. I am safe, free, and at peace. My favorite ways to experience quiet time with God is through prayer, reading (either the Bible or uplifting faith books), and through journaling, which brings me to mindfulness technique number five…

You can do three of these five techniques in one with journaling. You can practice gratitude, focus on God's presence, and have quiet time all through mindful journaling. Keeping a journal has been a part of my life for years, but I truly saw the difference in my outlook on life when I focused on God and gratitude as I wrote.

Things to Include in your Mindful Journal:
- All the positive things about the day (what you are grateful for)
- Written prayers or letters to God
- Any lessons you learned through either your experiences, reading, or Bible studies
- Any questions you have about life
- God moment stories: These are stories about when you notice God working in your life. One cool thing about taking the time to mindfully notice God's presence every day is that you...well... **notice** God's presence regularly.

Since I started mindfully taking the time to notice God in the present moment, I have had so many "goose-bump" God moments. These are those moments that I think, 'oh I will remember this,' but as time passes, I find I can't remember the details. Before including these God moment stories in my journal, I would remember *something* pretty cool happened, but I couldn't bring the vague memory to the surface in my mind.

By including these God moment stories in my journal, I solidify these events to my memory, and if I do forget, I can look at my journal and experience the awe and wonder all over again.

(P.S. You can find some of my "God Moment" stories on my "Inspiring Faith Stories" Pinterest Board)

6. Mindful Eating

As mentioned earlier, mindful eating is yet another time to pause from the day and focus on God, feel grateful, and enjoy a peaceful experience. When I mindfully focus on God's presence while eating, I do much less overeating. In fact, I like to say a little prayer before I eat.

As I pray, I think about 1 Corinthians 10:31 which says, "**So whether you eat or drink or whatever you do, do it all for the glory of God.**"

My prayer before I eat goes something like this, "God, thank you so much for this food. Thank you for this time that I have to sit and enjoy the food you have given me. I want to eat for the glory of You, God."

After saying this prayer, I enjoy my food, and I enjoy my time eating in God's presence.

And there you have it; six mindfulness exercises you can incorporate into your day.

A Step by Step Guide

Okay, let's take a moment to look at the specific techniques you can use to start mindfully eating. I want to give you a step-by-step guide to mindful eating because mindful eating has become a gift in my life, and I want you to have that gift too.

Step 1: Preparing your food

When preparing, avoid mindlLESSly nibbling while you are cooking. Instead focus on the joy of cooking. When you are stirring something in a bowl, focus simply on stirring.

Step 2: Plating your Food

When plating your food, be conscious of how much you are plating. PAUSE and ask yourself is this a reasonable amount of food? Do not starve yourself. Don't eat so little at one meal or throughout the day that you binge the next day. Just look and ask yourself is this a reasonable amount of food. Think about a healthy plate vs. an over-the-top plate. How does your plate compare?

Before sitting down, PAUSE to make sure you were not mindlessly piling on the food. Remember, pausing is the major piece to the Mindful eating process.

Step 3: Eating your Food

Remember to sit down and eat from a plate. Before putting a bite in your mouth, PAUSE. Really notice the food. Thank God for this time to enjoy your food. Think of this moment as a time to focus on God's presence and feel grateful. Say a prayer before you begin your eating experience. As I pray, I think about 1 Corinthians 10:31 which says, "So whether you eat or drink or whatever you do, do it all for the glory of God." Notice the color, textures, and smells before your first bite. Continue to do this for every bite. Put your fork down between each bite. Prepare the next bite after you have swallowed and taken a sip of drink. Take a sip of drink between each bite. During the meal, PAUSE occasionally to notice if you are full and ask yourself questions.

Ask questions like "Am I full?"; "How does this bite taste?"; "Am I enjoying my food?" "Am I hungry or emotionally eating?" Asking these questions helps you stay mindfully aware throughout the meal. You will be surprised at how full and satisfied you will be on the appropriate amount of food for your body. The key is pausing before you put food into your mouth. Listen to your body.

Step 4: Snacking on Food

Just like with a meal, PAUSE before and during the snack to ask yourself if you are mindfully snacking. Before putting a bite in your mouth, ask yourself "Is this mindLESS eating?" If the answer is 'yes', then save your food for when you can truly enjoy your food. No sense in wasting calories on food you are not enjoying. So are you mindLESSly snacking during cooking? Do you mindlessly grab store samples, or do lots of mindless nibbling at socials? Do you graze on leftovers during dinner clean up, or (my issue) eat cold toddler leftovers? If the answer is 'yes, I am mindlessly eating', then ask yourself why? Are you bored, stressed, or tired and wanting to eat even when you are not physically hungry? If you are not hungry, tell yourself you can wait until the next meal, which is only BLANK (insert the amount of time until your next meal) hours away. Usually you only have 30 minutes to 2 hours before the next meal. If you ask yourself the question, "Are you hungry?" and you are hungry, get a plate, sit down, and follow steps 1 through 3.

Step 5: Eating at Restaurants

Ask the waiter for a box as soon as your food arrives. Mindfully, fill the box with food from your plate until your plate looks like an appropriate meal so that you won't just mindlessly eat food just because it is there. Remember mindfulness is being aware of what you are doing at each moment. Be aware of what you are leaving on your plate. Then, follow step 3 to eat your food.

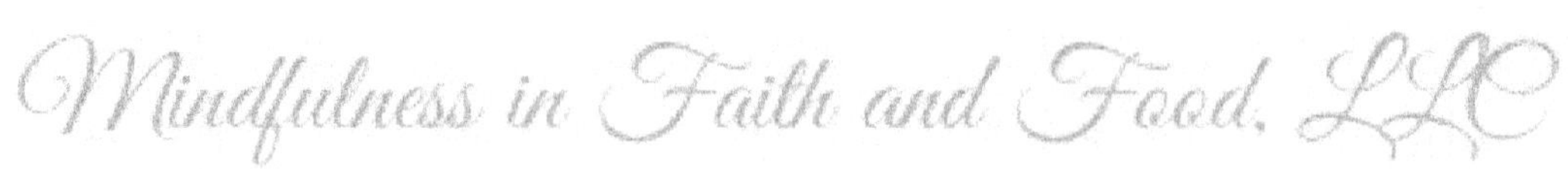

Thank you for purchasing The Nourishing Meal Builder!

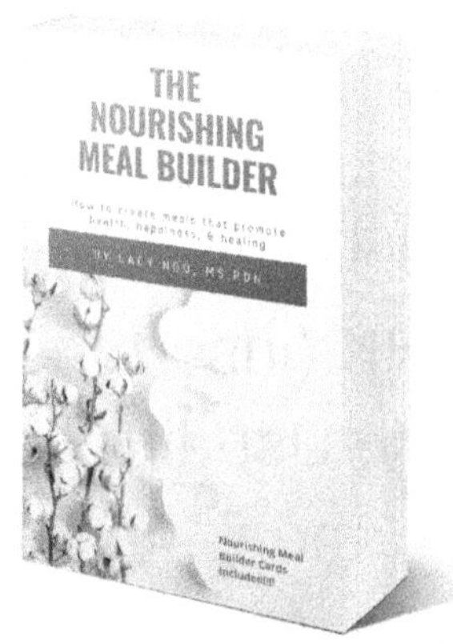

As a gift to you, here is a 25% off coupon code for any other Mindfulness in Faith and Food, LLC eboooks: THANKYOU25

You are also invited to become a member of the Mindful Family for FREE! You can join here!

As memebers, you will receive:

- The FREE 7-day Mindful Planner
- The FREE Random Acts of KIndness Planner
- The FREE Mindful Lunchbox Notes
- The FREE Healthy Lunchbox Checklist and More!

Selected References

Aragon G, Graham DB, Borum M, Doman DB. Probiotic Therapy for Irritable Bowel Syndrome. Gastroenterology & Hepatology. 2010;6(1):39-44.

Bhatia V., Tandon R., Stress and the Gastrointestinal Tract. Journal of Gastroenterology and Hepatology. 2005;20(3):332-339. doi:10.1111/j.1440-1746.2004.03508.x.

Bibiloni R, Fedorak R, Tannock G et al. VSL#3 Probiotic-Mixture Induces Remission in Patients with Active Ulcerative Colitis. The American Journal of Gastroenterology. 2005;100(7):1539-1546. doi:10.1111/j.1572-0241.2005.41794.x.

Bischoff S., Microbiota and aging. Current Opinion in Clinical Nutrition and Metabolic Care. 2016;19(1):26-30. doi:10.1097/mco.0000000000000242

Bischoff S.C., Barbara G., Buurman W., et al. Intestinal permeability – a new targetfor disease prevention and therapy. BMC Gastroenterology. 2014;14:189.doi:10.1186/s12876-014-0189-7.

Brahe L., Astrup A., Larsen L., Can We Prevent Obesity-Related Metabolic Diseases by Dietary Modulation of the Gut Microbiota?. Advances in Nutrition: An International Review Journal. 2016;7(1):90-101. doi:10.3945/an.115.010587.

Camilleri M., Madsen K., Spiller R., Van Meerveld B., Verne G., Intestinal barrier function in health and gastrointestinal disease. Neurogastroenterology & Motility. 2012;24(6):503-512. doi:10.1111/j.1365-2982.2012.01921.x.

Campbell A.W., Autoimmunity and the Gut. Autoimmune Diseases. 2014;2014:152428. doi:10.1155/2014/152428. Carabotti

Carabotti M., Scirocco A., Maselli M.A., Severi C., The gut-brain axis: interactions between enteric microbiota, central and enteric nervous systems. Annals of Gastroenterology : Quarterly Publication of the Hellenic Society of Gastroenterology. 2015;28(2):203-209.

Chassaing B., Koren O., Goodrich J., et al. Dietary emulsifiers impact the mouse gutmicrobiota promoting colitis and metabolic syndrome. Nature. 2015;519(7541):92-96.doi:10.1038/nature14232.

Ciorba M.A., A Gastroenterologist's Guide to Probiotics. Clinical gastroenterology and hepatology: the official clinical practice journal of the American Gastroenterological Association. 2012;10(9):960-968. doi:10.1016/j.cgh.2012.03.024.

Didari T., Effectiveness of probiotics in irritable bowel syndrome: Updated systematic review with meta-analysis. World Journal of Gastroenterology. 2015;21(10):3072. doi:10.3748/wjg.v21.i10.3072.

Distrutti E., Monaldi L., Ricci P., Fiorucci S., Gut microbiota role in irritable bowel syndrome: New therapeutic strategies. World Journal of Gastroenterology. 2016;22(7):2219-2241. doi:10.3748/wjg.v22.i7.2219.

DuPont H., Review article: evidence for the role of gut microbiota in irritable bowel syndrome and its potential influence on therapeutic targets. Alimentary Pharmacology & Therapeutics. 2014;39(10):1033-1042. doi:10.1111/apt.12728.
Eat

Farhadi A., Banan A., FIELDS J, Keshavarzian A. Intestinal barrier: An interface between health and disease. Journal of Gastroenterology and Hepatology. 2003;18(5):479-497. doi:10.1046/j.1440-1746.2003.03032.x.

Fasano A., Shea-Donohue T., Mechanisms of Disease: the role of intestinal barrier function in the pathogenesis of gastrointestinal autoimmune diseases. Nature Clinical Practice Gastroenterology & Hepatology. 2005;2(9):416-422. doi:10.1038/ncpgasthep0259.

Fasano A., Zonulin and Its Regulation of Intestinal Barrier Function: The Biological Door to Inflammation, Autoimmunity, and Cancer. Physiological Reviews. 2011;91(1):151-175. doi:10.1152/physrev.00003.2008.

Fond G., Boukouaci W., Chevalier G., et al. The "psychomicrobiotic": Targeting microbiota in major psychiatric disorders: A systematic review. Pathol Biol (Paris). 2015;63(1):35-42. doi: 10.1016/j.patbio.2014.10.003.

Forsythe P., Kunze W., Voices from within: gut microbes and the CNS. Cellular and Molecular Life Sciences. 2012;70(1):55-69. doi:10.1007/s00018-012-1028-z.

Hoban A. E., et al. (2016). Regulation of prefrontal cortex myelination by the microbiota. Transl. Psychiatry, doi: 10.1038/tp.2016.42.

Jangi S., Gandhi R., Cox L., et al. Alterations of the human gut microbiome in multiple sclerosis. Nat Commun. 2016;7.doi: 10.1038/ncomms12015.

Koloski N., Jones M, Kalantar J., Weltman M., Zaguirre J., Talley N., The brain–gut pathway in functional gastrointestinal disorders is bidirectional: a 12-year prospective population-based study. Gut. 2012;61(9):1284-1290. doi:10.1136/gutjnl-2011-300474.

Konturek P., Brzozowski T., Konturek S., Stress and the gut: pathophysiology, clinical consequences, diagnostic approach and treatment options. J Physiol Pharmacol. 2017;62(6):591-59.

Laird K., Tanner-Smith E., Russell A., Hollon S., Walker L., Comparative efficacy of psychological therapies for improving mental health and daily functioning in irritable bowel syndrome: A systematic review and meta-analysis. Clinical Psychology Review. 2017;51:142-152. doi:10.1016/j.cpr.2016.11.001.

Liu, R. T. (2017). The microbiome as a novel paradigm in studying stress and mental health. American Psychologist, 72(7), 655-667.http://dx.doi.org/10.1037/amp0000058

Logan A, Jacka F, Craig J, Prescott S. The Microbiome and Mental Health: Looking Back, Moving Forward with Lessons from Allergic Diseases. Clinical Psychopharmacology and Neuroscience. 2016;14(2):131-147. doi:10.9758/cpn.2016.14.2.131.

Maroon, Joseph. et al. Natural Anti-inflammatory agents for Pain Relief. Surg NeurolInt. 2010 Dec 13.

Mayer E, Knight R, Mazmanian S, Cryan J, Tillisch K. Gut Microbes and the Brain: Paradigm Shift in Neuroscience. Journal of Neuroscience. 2014;34(46):15490-15496. doi:10.1523/jneurosci.3299-14.2014.

Miele E, Pascarella F, Giannetti E, Quaglietta L, Baldassano R, Staiano A. Effect of a Probiotic Preparation (VSL#3) on Induction and Maintenance of Remission in Children With Ulcerative Colitis. The American Journal of Gastroenterology. 2009;104(2):437-443. doi:10.1038/ajg.2008.118.

Moayyedi P, Ford A, Talley N et al. The efficacy of probiotics in the treatment of irritable bowel syndrome: a systematic review. Gut. 2008;59(3):325-332.doi:10.1136/gut.2008.167270.

Moos W, Faller D, Harpp D et al. Microbiota and Neurological Disorders: A Gut Feeling. BioResearch Open Access. 2016;5(1):137-145. doi:10.1089/biores.2016.0010

Neuman H, Debelius J, Knight R, Koren O. Microbial endocrinology: the interplay between the microbiota and the endocrine system. FEMS Microbiology Reviews. 2015;39(4):509-521. doi:10.1093/femsre/fuu010.

Ojetti V, Ianiro G, Tortora A, D'Angelo G, et al. The Effect of Lactobacillus reuteri Supplementation in Adults with Chronic Functional Constipation: a Randomized, Double-Blind, Placebo-Controlled Trial. Journal of Gastrointestinal and Liver Diseases.2014;23(4). doi:10.15403/jgld.2014.1121.234.elr.

PaÅNrtty A, KalliomaÅNki M, Wacklin P, Salminen S, Isolauri E. A possible link between early probiotic intervention and the risk of neuropsychiatric disorders later in childhood: a randomized trial. Pediatric Research. 2015;77(6):823-828. doi:10.1038/pr.2015.51.

Rogers G, Keating D, Young R, Wong M, Licinio J, Wesselingh S. From gut dysbiosis to altered brain function and mental illness: mechanisms and pathways. Molecular Psychiatry. 2016;21(6):738-748. doi:10.1038/mp.2016.50.

Round JL, Mazmanian SK. The gut microbiome shapes intestinal immune responses during health and disease. Nature reviews Immunology. 2009;9(5):313-323. doi:10.1038/nri2515.

Sarkar A, Lehto S, Harty S, Dinan T, Cryan J, Burnet P. Psychobiotics and the Manipulation of Bacteria–Gut–Brain Signals. Trends in Neurosciences. 2016;39(11):763-781. doi:10.1016/j.tins.2016.09.002.

Scarlata, K. Overgrowth - What to Do When Unwelcome Microbes Invade. Today's Dietitian. 2011;13(4):46. Available at: http://www.todaysdietitian.com/newarchives/040511p46.shtml.

Stilling R, Dinan T, Cryan J. Microbial genes, brain & behavior - epigenetic regulation of the gut-brain axis. Genes, Brain and Behavior. 2013;13(1):69-86. doi:10.1111/gbb.12109.

Strati F, Cavalieri D, Albanese D et al. New evidences on the altered gut microbiota in autism spectrum disorders. Microbiome. 2017;5(1). doi:10.1186/s40168-017-0242-1.

Wasielewski H, Alcock J, Aktipis A. Resource conflict and cooperation between human host and gut microbiota: implications for nutrition and health. Annals of the New York Academy of Sciences. 2016;1372(1):20-28. doi:10.1111/nyas.13118.

Giancoli AN, Striving for Longevity. Today's Dietitian. 2017; 19 (5): 32.

Tufin AE, Bilici R, Usta G, Erdogan A. Mood disorder with mixed, psychotic features due to vitamin b12 deficiency in an adolescent: case report. Child Adolesc Psychiatry Ment Health. 2012; 6: 25. Published online 2012 Jun 22. doi: 10.1186/1753-2000-6-25

Morris, MC. "Nutritional determinants of cognitive aging and dementia." Proceedings of Nutrition Society. 2012: 1-13

Darmadi-Blackberry IML, Wahlqvist A, Kouris-Blazos, et al. "Legumes: the most important dietary predictor of survival in older people of different ethnicities." Asia Pacific Jouranl of Clinical Nutrition. 2004: 217-220

Shakersain BG, Santoni SC, Larsson, et al. "Prudent diet may attenuate the adverse effects of Western diet on cognitive decline." Alzheimer's & Dementia. 2016: 100-109

Bookheimer SYBA, Renner A, Ekstrom, et al. "Pomegranate juice augments memory and fMRI activity in middle-aged and older adults with mild memory complaints." Evidence-Based CAM. 2013. 946298.doi: 10.1155/2013/946298

Chen X, Huang Y, Cheng HG, "Lover intake of vegetables and legumes associated with cognitive decline among illiterate elderly Chines: A 3-year cohort study." The Journal of Nutrition, Health, & Aging. 2012. 549-552.

Devore EE, Kang JH, Breteler MM, et al. "Dietary intakes of berries and flavonoids in relation to cognitive decline. Annals of Neurology. 2012: 135-143.

Morris MC, Evans DA, Tangney A, et al. "Associations of vegetables and fruit with age-related cognitive change. Neurology. 2006: 1370-1376.

Martinez-Lapiscine EH, Clavero P, Toledo E, et al. "Mediterranean diet improves cognition: the PREDIMED-HAVARRA randomized trial." Journal of Neurology, Neurosurgery, and Psychiatry. 2013: 1318-1325.

Morris MC. "Nutritional determinants of cognitive again and dementia." Proceedings of Nutrition Society 2012: 1-13.

Morris MC, Tangney CC, Wang Y, et al. "MIND diet slows cognitive decline with aging." Alzheimer's &Dementia. 2015: 1015-1022

Barnard ND, Bush AI, Ceccarelli A, et a;. "Dietary and lifestyle guidelines for the prevention of Alzheimer's disease." Neurobiology of Aging. 2014: s74-s78.

Bes-Rastrollo M, Wedick NM, Martinez-Gonzalez MA, et al. "Prospective study of nut consumption, long-term weight change and obesity in women." The American Journal of Clinical Nutrition. 2009: 1913-1919.

Carey AN, Poulose SM, Shukitt-Hale B. "The beneficial effects of tree nuts on the aging brain." Nutrition and Aging. 2012: 55-67.

Valls-Pedret C, Sala-Vila A, Serra-Mir M, et al. "Mediterranean diet and age-related cognitive decline: a randomized clinical trial." JAMA Internal Medicine. 2015: 1094-1103.

Estuch R, Ros E, Salas-Salvado J, et al. "Primary prevention of cardiovascular disease with a Mediterranean diet." New England Journal of Medicine. 2013: 1279-1290.

Ptomey L, Steger FL, Schubert M, et al. "Breakfast intake and composition is associated with superior academic achievement in elementary school children." Journal of the American College of Nutrition. 2015: 1-8.

Peet M, "International Variations in the outcome of Schizophrenia and the Prevalence of Depression in Relation to National Dietary Practices: An Ecological Analysis." British Journal of Psychiatry. 2004. 184 (5) 404-408.

Sanchez A, Toledo E. "Fast-Food and commercial baked goods consumption and the risk of depression" Public Health Nutrition. 2012. (3) 15: 424-432.

Sanchez-Villegas A, Delgado-Rodriguez. M. "Association of the Mediterranean Dietary pattern with the incidence of depression." Archives of General Psychiatry. 2009 (10): 10990-1098.

Spedding S, "Vitamin D and depression: a systemic review and meta-analysis comparing studies with and without biological flaws." Nutrients. 2014. (4): 1501-1518.

Appleton KM, Rogers PJ, Ness AR. "Updated systemic review and meta-analysis of the effects of n-3 long-chain polyunsaturated fatty acids on depressed mood." American Journal of Clinical Nutrition. 2010. 91 (3): 757-770.

Bertone-Johnson ER, Powers SI, Spangler L, et al. "The Vitamin D intake from foods and supplements and depressive symptoms in a diverse population of older women" American Journal of Clinical Nutriton. 2011. 94 (4): 11-4-1112.

Grosso G. Pajak, Marventano. "Role of Omega-3 fatty acids in the treatment of depressive disorders: a comprehensive meta-analysis of randomized clinical trials. PLoS ONE. 2014. 9 (5): e96905.

Berick P, Denou E, Collins J, et al. "The intestinal microbiota affect central levels of brain-derived neurotropic factor and behavior in mice." Gastroenterology. 2011. 141 (2): 599-609. Doi: 10. 1053/j.gastro.2011.04.052.

Buydens-Branchey L, Branchey M, Hibbeln JR. "Association between increase in plasma N-3 poluunsaturated fatty acids following supplementation and decreases in anger and anxiety in substance abusers." Progress in Neuro-Psychopharmacology and Biological Psychiatry. 2008. 32 (2): 568-575. Doi:10.1016/j.pnpbp.2007.10.020.

Chorney DB, Detweiler F, Morris TL, et al. "The Interplay of sleep disturbance, anxiety, and depression in children. Journal of Pediatric Psychology. 2008. 33 (4): 339-348. Doi:10.1093/jpepsy/jsm105.

De Oliveira IJ, De Souza VV, Motta V, et al. "The effects of oral vitamin C supplementation on anxiety in students: a double-blind, randomized, placebo-controlled trial." Pakistan Journal of Biological Sciences. 2015. 18 (1): 11-18. Doi: 10.3923/pjbs.2015.11.18.

Kennedy DO. "B Vitamins and the brain: Mechanisms, dose, and efficacy- a review." Nutrients. 2016. 8 (2): 68. Doi: 10.3390/nu80068.

Kimura KM, Ozeki L, Juneja R, et al. "L-Theanine reduces psychological and physiological stress responses." Biological Psychology. 2007. 74 (1): 39-45. Doi: 10. 1016/j.biopsycho.2006.06.006.

Lakhan SE. Viera KF. Nutritional Therapies for mental disorders. Nutrition Journal. 2008, (2) doi:10.1186/1475-2891-7-2.

Maes M, Kubera M, Leunis JC. The gut-brain barrier in major depression: Intestinal Mucosal Dysfunction with an Increased translocation of LPS from Gram-negative Enterobacteria (Leaky Gut) plays a role in the inflammatory pathophysiology of depression. Neuro Endocrinology Letters. 2009, 29 (1): 117-124.

Pizzorno J. Glutathione! Integrative Medicine. 2014, 13 (1): 8-12.

Sartori SB, Whittle N, Hetzenauer, et al. Magnesium deficiency induces anxiety and HPA-axis dysregulation: Modulation by therapeutic drug treatment. Neuropharmacology. 2012, 62 (1): 304-312.

Selhub EM, Logan AC, Bested AC. Fermented foods, microbial, and mental health: ancient practice meets nutritional psychiatry. Journal of Physiological Anthropology. 2014, 33 (1): 2. Doi: 10.1186/1880-6805-33-2.

Wu A, Noble EE, Tyagi E, et al. Curcumin boosts DHA in the brain: implications for prevention of anxiety disorders. Biochimica et Biophysica Acta (BBA)- Molecular Basis of Disease 2015. 1852 (5): 951-961. Doi: 10.1016/j.bbadis.2014.12.005.

Aucoin M, Lalonde-Parsi M-J, Cooley K. Mindfulness-Based Therapies in the Treatment of Functional Gastrointestinal : A Meta-Analysis. Evidence-based Complementary and Alternative Medicine : eCAM. 2014;2014:140724. doi:10.1155/2014/140724.

Bakosh LS. Doctoral dissertation. 2013. Investigating the effects of a daily audio-guided mindfulness intervention for elementary school students and teachers. Available from ProQuest Dissertations & Theses database. (UMI No. 3618722)

Parker AE, Kupersmidt JB, Willoughby MT. An investigation of mindfulness education and self-regulation in middle school classrooms. 2014. Manuscript in preparation.

Black DS, Fernando R. Mindfulness training and classroom behavior among lower-income and ethnic minority elementary school children. Journal of Child and Family Studies. 2014;23:1242–1246. [PMC free article] [PubMed]

Bakosh LS, Snow RM, Tobias JM, Houlihan JL, Barbosa-Leiker C. Maximizing mindful learning: An innovative mindful awareness intervention improves elementary school students' quarterly grades. Mindfulness. 2015 Advance online publication.

Diamond A, Barnett WS, Thomas J, Munro S. Preschool program improves cognitive control. Science. 2007;318:1387–1388. [PMC free article] [PubMed]

Parker AE, Kupersmidt JB, Mathis ET, Scull TM, Sims C. The impact of mindfulness education on elementary school students: evaluation of the Master Mind program. Advances in School Mental Health Promotion. 2014;7:184–204. [PMC free article] [PubMed]

Britton WB, Lepp NE, Niles HF, Rocha T, Fisher NE, Gold JS. A randomized controlled pilot trial of classroom-based mindfulness meditation compared to an active control condition in sixth-grade children. Journal of School Psychology. 2014;52:263–278. http://doi.org/10.1016/j.jsp.2014.03.002. [PMC free article] [PubMed]

Hofmann SG, Sawyer AT, Witt AA, Oh D. The effect of mindfulness-based therapy on anxiety and depression: A meta-analytic review. Journal of Consulting and Clinical Psychology. 2010;78:169–183. [PMC free article] [PubMed]

Semple R, Droutman V, Reid BA. Mindfulness Goes to School: Things Learned (So Far) from Research and Real World Experiences. Psychol. Sch. 2017 Jan 54 (1): 29-52. https://www.ncbi.nlm.nih.gov/pmc/articles/PMC5405439/

Liu, R. T. (2017). The microbiome as a novel paradigm in studying stress and mental health. American Psychologist, 72(7), 655-667.http://dx.doi.org/10.1037/amp0000058

Mayer E, Knight R, Mazmanian S, Cryan J, Tillisch K. Gut Microbes and the Brain:Paradigm Shift in Neuroscience. Journal of Neuroscience. 2014;34(46):15490-15496. doi:10.1523/jneurosci.3299-14.2014.

Rogers G, Keating D, Young R, Wong M, Licinio J, Wesselingh S. From gut dysbiosis to altered brain function and mental illness: mechanisms and pathways. Molecular Psychiatry. 2016;21(6):738-748. doi:10.1038/mp.2016.50.

Bode A, Dong Z. The Amazing and Mighty Ginger. Herbal Medicine: The Bimolecular and Clinical Aspects. 2nd edition. 2011. 131-156. Doi:10.1201/b10787-8 Ginger

Butt MS, Pasha I, Sultan MT, Randhawa MA, Saeed F, Ahmed W. Black Pepper and Health Claims: A Comprehensive Treatise. Critical Reviews in Food Science and Nutrition. 2013. 53 (9) 875-886. Doi:10.1080/1040898.2011.571799.

Gupta SC, Patchva S, Aggarwal BB. Therapeutic roles of Curcumin: lessons learned from clinicial trails. The AAPS Journal. 2012. 15 (1) 195-218. Doi:10.1208/s12248-012-9432-8 Tumeric

Hewlings S, Kalman D. Curcumin: a review of its' effects on human health. Foods. 2017. 6(10) 92. Doi:10.3390/foods6100092 Tumeric

Jung-Chun L, Jeng-Shyan D, Chaun-Sung C, et al. Anti-inflammatory activities of Cinnamonum cassia constituents in vitro and in vivo. Evidence-Based Complementary and Alternative Medicine. 2012. 2012, http://dx.doi.org/10.1155/2012/429320

Miguel M, Antunes M, Faleiro M. Honey as a complementary medicine. Integrative Medicine Insights. 2017. 12, 117863371770286. Doi:10.1177/1178633717702869

Sahib NG, Anwar F, Gilani A, Hamid AA, Saari N, Alkharfy KM. Coriander: A potential source of high-value components for functional foods and nutraceuticals-a review. Phytotherapy Research. 2012. n/a-n/a. doi:10.1002/ptr.4897.

Yadav VS, Mishra KP, Singh DP, et al. Immunomodulatory effects of Curcumin. Immunopharmacology and Immunotoxicology. 2005. 27 (3), 485-497. Doi:10.1080/08923970500242244

Soundararajan, P, Gauri Junnarkar V, A Primer on Ayurveda: A Practical Guide on Personalized Nutrition for Dietitians, Nutritionists, and Healthcare Professionals. 2018. Ayur Wellness Inc DBA Ayurnutrition and Pushpa Soundararajan, RDN, LDN

Blessing EM, Steenkamp MM, Msnzanares J, et al. "Cannabidiol as a potential treatment for anxiety disorder.: Neurotherapeutics. 2015. 12 (4): 825-836 doi: 10.1007/s13311-015-0387-1

The Power of Positive Thinking. John Hopkins Medicine. https://www.hopkinsmedicine.org/health/healthy_aging/healthy_mind/the-power-of-positive-thinking

Positive Thinking: Stop Negative Self Talk to Reduce Stress. Mayo Clinic. 2017. https://www.mayoclinic.org/healthy-lifestyle/stress-management/in-depth/positive-thinking/art-20043950

Grotzkyj-Giorgi M. Nutrition and addiction- can dietary changes assist with recovery? Drug and Alcohol Today. 2009, 9 (2) 24-28.

Salz A. CPE Monthly: Substance Abuse and Nutrition. Today's Dietitan. 2014, 16 (12): 44.

Melo K. Simply Fresh: Health Made Simple. 2017. Typo Fire.

Haugen M, Cook D. 175 Superfood Blender Recipes Using your NutriBullet. 2017. Robert Rose Inc.

Miller A. The Anti-anxiety Diet. 2018. Ulysses Press.

Mood M. The Mind Diet. 2016. Ulysses Press.

Babb M. Anti-inflammatory Eating for a Happy, Healthy Brain. 2016. Sasquatch Books.

Soundararajan P, Junnarkar VG. A Primer on Ayurveda: A Practical Guide on Personalized Nutrition for Dietitians, Nutritionists, & Healthcare Professionals. 2018.

Rishikof D. Health Takes Guts: Your Comprehensive Guide to Eliminating Digestive Problems, Anxiety, & Fatigue. 2018.

Lydon K. Nourish your Namaste: How Nutrition and Yoga can Support Digestion, Immunity, Energy, & Relaxation.

Giugliano D, Ceriello A, Esposito K. The Effects of Diet on Inflammation. Journal of the American College of Cardiology. 2006. DOI: 10.1016/j.jacc.2006.03.052